Anxiety

by Charles H. Elliott, PhD
Laura L. Smith, PhD

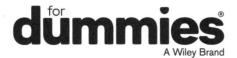

Anxiety For Dummies®

Published by: **John Wiley & Sons, Inc.,** 111 River Street, Hoboken, NJ 07030-5774, www.wiley.com

Copyright © 2021 by John Wiley & Sons, Inc., Hoboken, New Jersey

Published simultaneously in Canada

For general information on our other products and services, please contact our Customer Care Department within the U.S. at 877-762-2974, outside the U.S. at 317-572-3993, or fax 317-572-4002. For technical support, please visit https://hub.wiley.com/community/support/dummies.

Wiley publishes in a variety of print and electronic formats and by print-on-demand. Some material included with standard print versions of this book may not be included in e-books or in print-on-demand. If this book refers to media such as a CD or DVD that is not included in the version you purchased, you may download this material at http://booksupport.wiley.com. For more information about Wiley products, visit www.wiley.com.

Library of Congress Control Number: 2020949876

ISBN 978-1-119-76850-0 (pbk); ISBN 978-1-119-76856-2 (ebk); ISBN 978-1-119-76853-1 (ebk)

Manufactured in the United States of America

SKY10022858_112520

Contents at a Glance

Table of Contents

Introduction

We wrote our first book in the *For Dummies* series, *Overcoming Anxiety For Dummies,* shortly after the events of 9-11-2001. People felt rather anxious, especially about terrorism. We wrote the second edition in 2010 as the Great Recession was winding down. At that time, people were feeling particularly anxious about their finances and careers. Today, we present *Anxiety For Dummies* as the world struggles to cope with a global pandemic, an explosion of civil unrest and racism, climate change, and another potentially massive recession or depression.

So today's world, just like the previous two decades, gives us plenty to worry about. But as we don't want to become victims of a pandemic, financial setback, natural disaster, or violence, we can't let ourselves become victims of anxiety. Anxiety clouds our thinking and weakens our resolve to live life to the fullest. We realize that some anxiety is realistic and inescapable, yet, we can keep it from dominating our lives. Even under duress, we can preserve a degree of serenity; we can hold onto our humanity, vigor, and zest for life. We can love and laugh.

Because we believe in our collective resilience, we take a humorous, and at times irreverent, approach to conquering anxiety. Our message is based on sound, scientifically proven methods. But we don't bore you with the scientific details. Instead, we present a clear, rapid-fire set of strategies for beating back anxiety and winning the war against worry.

About This Book

We have three goals in writing this book. First, we want you to understand just what anxiety is and some of the different forms it can take. Second, we think that knowing what's good about anxiety and what's bad about it is useful for you. Finally, we cover what you're probably most interested in — discovering the latest techniques for overcoming your anxiety and helping someone you care about who has anxiety.

Unlike most books, you don't have to start on page 1 and read straight through. Use the extensive table of contents to pick and choose what you want to read.

Don't worry about reading parts in any particular order. For example, if you really don't want much information about the who, what, when, where, and why of anxiety and whether you have it, go ahead and skip Part 1. However, we encourage you to at least skim Part 1, because it contains fascinating facts and information as well as ideas for getting started.

Scattered throughout this book are case examples and stories that illustrate important principles and techniques. Although these examples are based on composites of real people, they do not represent any actual person. Any similarities to actual cases or people are purely coincidental.

Foolish Assumptions

Who might pick up this book? We assume, probably foolishly, that you or someone you love suffers from some type of problem with anxiety or worry. But, it's also possible that you simply find the topic of anxiety interesting. We imagine that you may be curious about a variety of helpful strategies to choose from that can fit your lifestyle and personality. Finally, you may be a mental health professional who's interested in finding a friendly resource for your clients who suffer from anxiety or worry.

Icons Used in This Book

For Dummies books use little pictures, called *icons,* in the margins to get your attention. Here's what they mean:

REMEMBER

The Remember icon appears when we want your attention. Please read the text associated with it for critical information.

TIP

The Tip icon alerts you to important insights, clarifications, or ways to do things better.

WARNING

Warning icons appear when you need to be careful, avoid potential risks, or seek professional help.

The Technical Stuff icon highlights information that some readers will find interesting but is not necessary for your overall understanding of anxiety.

TECHNICAL STUFF

Beyond the Book

For quick tips about anxiety, go to www.dummies.com, and type "Anxiety For Dummies Cheat Sheet" in the search box. You can get information about how to identify anxious thoughts, behaviors, and feelings. In addition, there are some suggestions for dealing with your anxious symptoms.

Where to Go from Here

Anxiety For Dummies offers you the best, most up-to-date advice based on scientific research on anxiety disorders. If you want help controlling your negative thoughts, turn to Chapters 6 and 7. If you're concerned about living well during a pandemic, check out Chapter 13. If you're worried about your job and finances, in Chapter 14 we provide tips for finding your next job and pinching pennies. Chapter 16 is a new chapter about anxiety related to racism.

For some people, this book could be a complete guide to fighting frenzy and fear. However, some stubborn forms of anxiety need more care and attention. If your anxiety and worry significantly get in the way of work or play, get help. Start with your family doctor to rule out physical causes. Then, consult with a mental health professional. Anxiety can be conquered, so don't give up.

1

Detecting and Exposing Anxiety

Chapter **1**

Analyzing and Attacking Anxiety

S troll down the street and about one in four of the people you walk by has significant problems with anxiety. And almost half of the people you encounter will struggle with anxiety to one degree or another. The rate of anxiety across the world has climbed for many decades, and no end is in sight.

The whole world watches on edge as disasters, terrorism, financial collapse, pandemics, social unrest, crime, and war threaten the security of home and family. Anxiety creates havoc in the home, destroys relationships, erodes health, causes employees to lose time from work, and prevents people from living full, productive lives.

In this chapter, you find out how to recognize the signs and symptoms of anxiety. We clarify the costs of anxiety — both personal and societal. We provide a brief overview of the treatments presented in greater detail in later chapters. You also get a glimpse of how to help if someone you care about or your child has anxiety. If you worry too much, or care for someone who has serious problems with anxiety, this book is here to help!

Anxiety: Everybody's Doing It

Anxiety involves feelings of uneasiness, worry, apprehension, and/or fear, and it's the most common of all the emotional disorders. In other words, you definitely aren't alone if you have unwanted anxiety. And the numbers have grown over the years. At no time in history has anxiety tormented more people than it does today. Why?

Life has always been menacing. But today people around the world are glued to screens watching the latest horrors in real time. News feeds, blogs, tweets, newsprint, and social media chronicle crime, war, disease, discrimination, and corruption. The media's portrayal of these modern plagues includes full-color images with unprecedented, graphic clarity.

In addition, recurring financial crises rock the fragile stability of the poor as well as the middle class. The lack of basic necessities like food, shelter, education, healthcare, clean water, and sanitation endanger many lives throughout the world. No wonder anxiety is its own worldwide pandemic.

Unfortunately, as stressful and anxiety-arousing as the world is today, only a minority of those suffering from anxiety seek professional treatment. That's a problem, because anxiety causes not only emotional pain and distress but also physical strain and even death, given that anxiety extracts a serious toll on the body and sometimes even contributes to suicide. Furthermore, anxiety costs society as a whole, to the tune of billions of dollars.

When people talk about what anxiety feels like, you may hear any or all of the following descriptions:

>> When my panic attacks begin, I feel tightness in my chest. It's as though I'm drowning or suffocating, and I begin to sweat; the fear is overwhelming. I feel like I'm going to die, and I have to sit down because I may faint.

>> I've always been painfully shy. I want friends, but I'm too embarrassed to call anyone. I guess I feel like anyone I call will think I'm not worth talking to. I feel really lonely, but I can't even think about reaching out. It's just too risky.

> **»** I wake with worry every day, even on the weekends. Ever since I lost my job, I worry all the time. Sometimes, when it's really bad, I feel like I'm going crazy, and I can't even sleep.

> **»** I'm so afraid of everything that I can barely leave the house. I've stopped even looking for jobs. My family has to bring me groceries.

As you can see, anxiety results in all sorts of thoughts, behaviors, and feelings. When your anxiety begins to interfere with day-to-day life, you need to find ways to put your fears and worries at ease.

Tabulating the Costs of Anxiety

Anxiety costs. It costs the sufferer in emotional, physical, and financial terms. But it doesn't stop there. Anxiety also incurs a financial burden for everyone. Stress, worry, and anxiety disrupt relationships, work, and family.

THE HEARTBREAK OF ANXIETY

Cardiovascular disease stands as the number one cause of death throughout the world. And research has demonstrated that chronic anxiety is a major contributor to poor cardiac health. So, early diagnosis and treatment for anxiety may help prevent some heart disease.

When patients are diagnosed with heart disease, anxiety often increases, even among people without a history of anxiety. Numerous studies have shown that untreated anxiety among cardiac patients is linked to poorer outcomes. These poor outcomes include recurrent cardiac events and even higher rates of death.

Therefore, it's been recommended that all cardiac patients should be assessed for the presence of problems with anxiety. Since anxiety can be successfully treated, it makes sense to include evaluation and treatment for anxiety when it occurs in cardiac patients. Such interventions are likely to alleviate anxiety as well as contribute to improved cardiovascular health, but further research is needed to firmly establish this relationship.

What does anxiety cost you?

Obviously, if you have a problem with anxiety, you experience the cost of distressed, anxious feelings. Anxiety feels lousy. You don't need to read a book to know that. But did you know that untreated anxiety runs up a tab in other ways as well? These costs include

- >> **A physical toll:** Higher blood pressure, tension headaches, and gastrointestinal symptoms can affect your body. In fact, recent research found that certain types of chronic anxiety disorders change the makeup of your brain's structures.

- >> **A toll on your kids:** Parents with anxiety more often have anxious children. This is due in part to genetics, but it's also because kids learn from observation. Anxious kids may be so stressed that they can't pay attention in school.

- >> **Fat:** Anxiety and stress increase the stress hormone known as cortisol. Cortisol causes fat storage in the abdominal area, thus increasing the risk of heart disease and stroke. Stress also leads to increased eating.

- >> **More trips to the doctor:** That's because those with anxiety frequently experience worrisome physical symptoms. In addition, anxious people often worry a great deal about their health.

- >> **Relationship problems:** People with anxiety frequently feel irritable. Sometimes, they withdraw emotionally or do the opposite and dependently cling to their partners.

- >> **Downtime:** Those with anxiety disorders miss work more often than other people, usually as an effort to temporarily quell their distress.

The cost to society

Anxiety costs hundreds of billions of dollars worldwide each year. Most of the cost is due to loss of productivity. Decreased productivity is sometimes due to health problems made worse by anxiety. But the financial loss from downtime and healthcare costs doesn't include the dollars lost to substance abuse, which many of those with anxiety disorders turn to in order to deal with their anxiety. Thus, directly and indirectly, anxiety extracts a colossal toll on both the person who experiences it and society at large.

Recognizing the Symptoms of Anxiety

You may not know if you suffer from problematic anxiety. That's because anxiety involves a wide range of symptoms. Each person experiences a slightly different constellation of these symptoms. For now, you should know that some signs of anxiety appear in the form of thoughts or beliefs. Other indications of anxiety manifest themselves in bodily sensations. Still other symptoms show up in various kinds of anxious behaviors. Some people experience anxiety signs in all three ways, while others only perceive their anxiety in one or two areas.

Thinking anxiously

Folks with anxiety generally think in ways that differ from the ways that other people think. You're probably thinking anxiously if you experience:

>> **Approval addiction:** If you're an approval addict, you worry a great deal about what other people think about you.

>> **Living in the future and predicting the worst:** When you do this, you think about everything that lies ahead and assume the worst possible outcome.

>> **Dependency:** Some people believe they must have help from others and are unable to achieve on their own.

>> **Perfectionism:** If you're a perfectionist, you assume that any mistake means total failure.

>> **Poor concentration:** Anxious people routinely report that they struggle with focusing their thoughts. Short-term memory sometimes suffers as well.

>> **Racing thoughts:** Thoughts zip through your mind in a stream of almost uncontrollable worry and concern.

We discuss anxious thinking in great detail in Chapters 5, 6, and 7.

Behaving anxiously

We have three words to describe anxious behavior — avoidance, avoidance, and avoidance. Anxious people inevitably attempt to stay away from the things that make them anxious. Whether it's snakes, heights, crowds, freeways, parties, paying bills, reminders of bad times, or public speaking, anxious people search for ways out.

In the short run, avoidance lowers anxiety. It makes you feel a little better. However, in the long run, avoidance actually maintains and heightens anxiety. We give you ways of confronting avoidance in Chapter 9.

One of the most common and obvious examples of anxiety-induced avoidance is how people react to their phobias. Have you ever seen the response of a spider phobic when confronting one of the critters? Usually, such folks scream, jump, and hastily retreat.

Finding anxiety in your body

Almost all people with severe anxiety experience a range of physical effects. These sensations don't simply occur in your head; they're as real as this book you're holding. The responses to anxiety vary considerably from person to person and include the following:

>> Accelerated heartbeat

>> Shallow, rapid breathing

>> A spike in blood pressure

>> Dizziness

>> Fatigue

>> Gastrointestinal upset

>> General aches and pains

>> Muscle tension or spasms

>> Sweating

WARNING

These are simply the temporary effects that anxiety exerts on your body. Chronic anxiety left untreated poses serious risks to your health as well. We discuss the general health effects in greater detail in Chapter 2.

NAME THAT PHOBIA!

Phobias are one of the most common types of anxiety, and we discuss them in detail in Chapter 2. A *phobia* is an excessive, disproportionate fear of a relatively harmless situation or thing. Sometimes, the object of the phobia poses some risk, but the person's reaction clearly exceeds the danger. Do you know the technical names for phobias? Draw arrows from the common name of each phobia to the corresponding technical name. See how many you get right. The answers are printed upside down at the bottom.

Be careful if you have *triskaidekaphobia* (fear of the number 13), because we're giving you 13 phobias to match!

Technical Name	Means a Fear of This
1. Ophidiophobia	A. Growing old
2. Zoophobia	B. Sleep
3. Gerascophobia	C. The mind
4. Acrophobia	D. Imperfection
5. Lachanophobia	E. Snakes
6. Hypnophobia	F. Fear
7. Atealophobia	G. New things
8. Phobophobia	H. Animals
9. Sesquipedalophobia	I. Small things
10. Neophobia	J. Mirrors
11. Psychophobia	K. Heights
12. Microphobia	L. Long words
13. Eisoptrophobia	M. Vegetables

Answers:

1.	2.	3.	4.	5.	6.	7.	8.	9.	10.	11.	12.	13.
E,	H,	A,	K,	M,	B,	D,	F,	L,	G,	C,	I,	J

Seeking Help for Your Anxiety

As we say earlier in this chapter, most people simply choose to live with anxiety rather than seek professional help. Some people worry that treatment won't work. Or they believe that the only effective treatment out there is medication, and they fear the possibility of side effects. Others fret about the costs of getting help. And still others have concerns that tackling their anxiety would cause their fears to increase so much that they wouldn't be able to stand it.

TIP

Well, stop adding worry to worry. You can significantly reduce your anxiety through a variety of interesting strategies. Many of these don't have to cost a single cent. And if one doesn't work, you can try another. Most people find that at least a couple of the approaches that we review work for them. The following sections provide an overview of treatment options and give you some guidance on what to do if your self-help efforts fall short.

WARNING

Untreated anxiety may cause long-term health problems. It doesn't make sense to avoid doing something about your anxiety.

Matching symptoms and therapies

Anxiety symptoms appear in three different spheres, as follows (see the earlier section "Recognizing the Symptoms of Anxiety" for more details on these symptoms):

>> **Thinking symptoms:** The thoughts that run through your mind

>> **Behaving symptoms:** The things you do in response to anxiety

>> **Feeling symptoms:** How your body reacts to anxiety

Treatment corresponds to each of these three areas, as we discuss in the following three sections.

Thinking therapies

One of the most effective treatments for a wide range of emotional problems, known as *cognitive therapy,* deals with the way you think about, perceive, and interpret everything that's important to you, including

>> Your views about yourself

>> The events that happen to you in life

>> Your future

When people feel unusually anxious and worried, they almost inevitably distort the way they think about these things. That distortion actually causes much of their anxiety. In the following example, Luann has both physical symptoms and cognitive symptoms of anxiety. Her therapist chooses a cognitive approach to help her.

> Luann, a junior in college, gets physically ill before every exam. She throws up, has diarrhea, and her heart races. She fantasizes that she will fail each and every test she takes and that eventually, the college will dismiss her. Yet, her lowest grade to date has been a B–.

> The cognitive approach her therapist uses helps her capture the negative predictions and catastrophic outcomes that run through her mind. It then guides her to search for evidence about her true performance and a more realistic appraisal of the chances of her actually failing.

As simple as this approach sounds, hundreds of studies have found that it works well to reduce anxiety. Part 2 of this book describes various cognitive or thinking therapy techniques.

Behaving therapies

Another highly effective type of therapy is known as *behavior therapy.* As the name suggests, this approach deals with actions you can take and behaviors you can incorporate to alleviate your anxiety. Some actions are fairly straightforward, like getting more exercise and sleep and managing your responsibilities. You can get good ideas on those actions in Chapter 11.

On the other hand, a more critical type of action targets anxiety directly. It's called *exposure* and feels a little scary. Exposure involves breaking your fears down into small steps and facing them one at a time. We cover exposure in Chapter 9.

Some people, with the advice of their doctor, choose to take medications for their anxiety. If you're considering that option, be sure to see Chapter 10 to help you make an informed decision.

Feeling therapies: Soothing the inner storm

Anxiety sets off a storm of distressing physical symptoms, such as a racing heartbeat, upset stomach, muscle tension, sweating, dizziness, and so on. Making a few tweaks to your lifestyle such as increased exercise, better diet, and adequate sleep help a little. But our primary recommendation is to figure out how to approach distressing physical symptoms with an accepting attitude. Chapter 8 offers guidance on what's called mindful acceptance.

Finding the right help

We suppose it's not too presumptuous to assume that because you're reading this book, you or someone you know suffers from anxiety. And you'd probably like to tackle anxiety. This book is a great place to get started on managing your anxiety.

TIP

The good news is that a number of studies support the idea that people can deal with important, difficult problems without seeking the services of a professional. People clearly benefit from self-help. They get better and stay better.

Then again, sometimes self-help efforts fall short, especially when anxiety is moderate to severe in intensity. Chapter 23 provides ten critical signs that indicate a likely need for professional help. See Chapter 4 for information about finding the right professional for you.

If you do need professional consultation, many qualified therapists will work with you on the ideas contained in this book. That's because most mental health professionals will appreciate the comprehensive nature of the material and the fact that most of the strategies are based on well-proven methods. If research has yet to support the value of a particular approach, we take care to let you know that. We happen to think you're much better off sticking with strategies known to work and avoiding those that don't.

In Chapters 18, 19, and 20, we discuss how to help a child or an adult loved one who has anxiety. If you're working with a friend or family member, you both may want to read Part 5, and probably more, of this book. Sometimes, friends and family can help those who are also working with a professional and making their own efforts.

Whichever sources, techniques, or strategies you select, overcoming anxiety will be one of the most rewarding challenges that you ever undertake. The endeavor may scare you at first, and the going may start slow and have its ups and downs. But if you stick with it, we believe that you'll find a way out of the quicksand of anxiety and onto the solid ground of acceptance.

Chapter **2**

Examining What Anxiety Is All About

Anxious feelings sprout up for most folks here and there and are completely normal. In certain situations, anxiety is a perfectly understandable reaction. For example, if you're driving in a snowstorm and your car starts to spin out of control, feeling anxious makes sense. Or, if you are in the middle of a pandemic and the numbers of infections keep rising, well, if you didn't feel a bit anxious, we'd worry about you. But sometimes anxiety signals something more serious. When anxiety is not tightly connected to realistic concerns and interferes with your ability to function day to day, it's a good time to worry about your anxiety.

To get a feel for the difference between something as serious as an anxiety disorder and a normal reaction, read the following description and imagine ten minutes in the life of Viktoria.

> **Viktoria** feels restless and shifts her weight from foot to foot. Walking forward a little, she notices a slight tightening in her chest. Her breathing quickens. She feels an odd mixture of excitement and mounting tension. She sits down and does her best to relax, but the anxiety continues to intensify. Her body suddenly jerks forward; she grips the sides of her seat and clenches her teeth to choke back a scream. Her stomach feels like it might come up through her throat. She feels her heart race and her face flush. Tiffany's emotions run wild. Dizziness, fear, and a rushing sensation overtake her. The feelings all come in waves — one after the other.

You may wonder what's wrong with poor Viktoria. Maybe she has an anxiety disorder. Or possibly she's suffering a nervous breakdown. Perhaps she's going crazy. No, Viktoria actually *wanted* to feel scared and anxious!

You see, she was at an amusement park. She handed her ticket to the attendant and buckled herself into a roller coaster. After that, you probably understand the rest of her experience. Viktoria doesn't have a problem with anxiety, she isn't suffering a nervous breakdown, and she isn't going crazy. As her story illustrates, the symptoms of anxiety can be ordinary and sometimes even desired reactions to life.

In this chapter, we help you figure out whether you're suffering from problematic anxiety, everyday anxiety, or something else. We take a close look at all the different forms and symptoms of anxiety. Then, we discuss some of the other emotional disorders that often accompany anxiety.

REMEMBER

Mental health professionals refer to emotional problems as disorders. For example, instead of saying you're depressed, they say you have a depressive disorder or some other type of mood disorder. A reasonable case can be made for using the term "disorder." Although we use the word from time to time, we prefer to think of so-called disorders as normal reactions to a combination of biological, genetic, environmental, and interpersonal factors, as well as learned behaviors and problematic thoughts.

Anxiety: Help or Hindrance?

Imagine a life with no anxiety at all. How wonderful! You wake up every morning anticipating nothing but pleasant experiences. You fear nothing. The future holds only sweet security and joy.

Think again. With no anxiety, when the guy in the car in front of you slams on the brakes, your response will be slower because your body doesn't react quickly to danger, and you'll be more likely to crash. With no worries about the future, your retirement may end up bleak because your lack of worry caused you to not save for the future. The total absence of anxiety may cause you to walk into a work presentation unprepared or not bother studying for an important test.

Anxiety is good for you! It prepares you to take action. It mobilizes your body for emergencies. It warns you about danger. Be *glad* you have some anxiety. Your anxiety helps you stay out of trouble. See the sidebar "Anxiety and driving while Black" for suggestions about how normal anxiety may help protect young Black drivers.

ANXIETY AND DRIVING WHILE BLACK

All parents of teenagers who are learning to drive are anxious. If you've ever been in the car with a brand-new driver, you understand what we're talking about. When the teen finally gets a license, the fear persists for some months. Will my daughter remember to stop at stop signs or make a turn without crashing into the curb? Will my son speed or try to show off while driving with his friends?

But if you are a parent of a Black teen driver (especially males), your worries multiply. Will my son be pulled over and know exactly what to say and do? What do I tell him to help him stay safe? Though it isn't fair or reasonable, parents of Black teens have to give "the talk." Usually the talk contains a few important elements that are useful for most people who get pulled over, but essential for persons of color. Here are a few items that usually get covered in the talk:

- While the officer approaches the car, roll down the window, turn off the ignition, and place your hands at the top of the steering wheel.

- Don't move your hands unless instructed to do so.

- When asked for license and registration, move slowly and tell the officer what you are doing, especially if you need to access the glove compartment.

- Be polite and cooperate.

- Do what the officer asks.

- It's not a good idea to argue or be defensive.

- Do not run or resist arrest.

- Don't make statements about what did or did not happen until you can talk to an attorney.

Again, it's unfair that people of color must take greater care during police encounters than others. But statistics tell us that persons of color have a greater chance of being hurt or killed at a traffic stop. This is a time when a good dose of anxiety may save a life.

REMEMBER

Anxiety poses a problem for you when

>> **It lasts uncomfortably long or occurs too often.** For example, if you have disturbing levels of anxiety most days for more than a few weeks, you have reason for concern.

>> **It interferes with doing what you want to do.** Thus, if anxiety wakes you up at night, causes you to make mistakes at work, or keeps you from going where you want to go, it's getting in the way.

>> **It exceeds the level of actual danger or risk.** For example, if your body and mind feel like an avalanche is about to bury you but all you're doing is taking a test for school, your anxiety has gone too far.

>> **You struggle to control your worries, but they keep on coming.** Even when you're relaxing at the beach or on your most comfortable recliner, anxious thoughts continually run through your mind.

What Anxiety Looks Like

Anxiety comes in various forms. The word "anxious" is a derivative of the Latin word *angere*, meaning to strangle or choke. A sense of choking or tightening in the throat or chest is a common symptom of anxiety. However, anxiety also involves other symptoms, such as sweating, trembling, nausea, and a racing heartbeat. Anxiety may also involve fears — fear of losing control and fear of illness or dying. In addition, people with excessive anxiety avoid various situations, people, animals, or objects to an unnecessary degree.

Anxious people tend to be extremely sensitive to danger, rejection, the unknown, and uncertainty. They may pay close attention to unpleasant thoughts, feelings, and physical sensations. They also often dwell on the possibility of future calamities. Anxiety symptoms such as these have a tendency to cluster together. The following sections describe some of these major clusters.

TECHNICAL STUFF

The following subheadings roughly correspond to some of the major diagnoses discussed in DSM-5, but we think it's more productive to focus on symptoms rather than technical diagnostic categories. (See the sidebar "The Diagnostic and Statistical Manual-5 [DSM-5]" for more information.)

Worrywarts

Most people have heard of the term "worrywart" and immediately conjure up someone who constantly worries. Worrywarts have a chronic state of tension and worry. They often report feeling restless, on edge, and keyed up. They may tire easily and have trouble concentrating or falling asleep. Once asleep, they may wake up at 3 a.m. with racing, worried thoughts. Worriers also often report having achy muscles, especially in the back, shoulders, or neck.

Not everyone experiences chronic worries in exactly the same way. Some worriers complain about other problems — such as twitching, trembling, shortness of breath, sweating, dry mouth, stomach upset, feeling shaky, being easily startled, and having difficulty swallowing. No matter how you experience worry, if it's keeping you from living life the way you want to, it's a problem.

The following profile offers an example of what excessive worry looks like.

> In a subway, **Brian** taps his foot nervously. He slept only a few hours last night, tossing, turning, and ruminating about the economy. He's sure that he's next in line to lose his job. Even though his boss says that he's safe, Brian can't stop worrying. He believes that he may end up broke and homeless.
>
> His back is killing him; he shrugs his shoulders trying to loosen up his tight muscles. He struggles to concentrate on the blog that he's looking at and realizes that he can't remember what he just read. He notices his shirt feels damp. He thinks he might be sick. He *is* sick — with worry.
>
> Brian has worked steadily at the same company since graduating from college six years ago. His work is highly technical. Most of the senior executives depend on his technology know-how. He has stashed away a nice amount of money for emergencies. Nevertheless, his anxiety has increased over the last year to the point that he notices that he's making mistakes. He can't think; he feels horrible and is in a constant state of distress.

The economy can make anyone anxious at times. But Brian's worries appear to be out of proportion to his real situation. It seems unlikely that he's in danger of losing his job. However, his extreme anxiety may, in fact, cause him to get in trouble at work. People with overwhelming anxiety often make careless mistakes because of problems with attention and concentration.

TIP

Some worries are perfectly normal. If you lose your job, it's quite natural to worry about money. But if your name is Bill Gates or Jeff Bezos and you're worried about money, perhaps you have a problem with anxiety.

TECHNICAL STUFF

When we were writing this section, we wondered where the original phrase "worrywart" came from. So, we looked it up. Turns out that Worry Wart was a character in a comic strip from the 1920s. The boy was a constant pest and annoyed his brother who christened him with the name Worry Wart. The meaning evolved into someone who is constantly beset with worries. The reason the word "wart" was used is that warts are an itchy nuisance that can't be scratched away. In fact, the more you scratch, the worse the wart becomes, a bit like worry.

Avoiding people

People who are socially phobic fear exposure to public scrutiny. These people dread performing, speaking, going to parties, meeting new people, entering groups, using the telephone, writing a check in front of others, eating in public, and/or interacting with those in authority. They see these situations as painful because they expect to receive humiliating or shameful judgments from others.

Social phobics believe they're somehow defective and inadequate; they assume they'll bungle their lines, spill their drinks, shake hands with clammy palms, or commit any number of social faux pas and thus embarrass themselves. Ironically, because they are so anxious, they actually do what they fear. Shaky, sweaty hands spill drinks. Lack of eye contact turns people away. They worry about what others are thinking about them — so much that they don't listen well enough to keep a conversation going.

REMEMBER

Everyone feels uncomfortable or nervous from time to time, especially in new situations. For example, if you've been experiencing social fears about a challenging new situation, that may be normal. A short-term fear of socializing may be a temporary reaction to a new stress such as moving to a new neighborhood or getting a new job. However, you may have a problem with social anxiety if you experience the following symptoms for a prolonged period:

>> You fear situations with unfamiliar people or ones where you may be observed or evaluated in some way.

>> When forced into an uncomfortable social situation, your anxiety increases powerfully. For example, if you fear public speaking, your voice shakes, and your knees tremble the moment that you start your speech.

>> You realize that your fear is greater than the situation really warrants. For example, if you fear meeting new people, logically you know nothing horrible will happen, but tidal waves of adrenaline and fearful anticipation course through your veins.

>> You avoid fearful situations as much as you can or endure them only with great distress. Because of your fears, you may miss a variety of events you'd otherwise like to go to (for example, family gatherings, work opportunities, or parties).

Check out the following prime example of a social anxiety and see whether any of it seems familiar.

Maurice, a 35-year-old bachelor, wants a serious relationship. Women consider him attractive, and he has a well-paying job. Maurice's friends invite him to parties and other social events in an effort to set him up with women. Unfortunately, he detests the idea of going. Maurice conjures up a number of good excuses for backing out. However, his desire to meet potential dates eventually wins.

Whenever he imagines scenes of meeting women, he feels intense, anxious anticipation.

When Maurice arrives at the party, he heads to the bar to quell his mounting anxiety. His hands shake as he picks up his first drink. Quickly downing the drink, he orders another in hopes of numbing his emotions. After an hour of nonstop drinking, he feels much braver. He interrupts a cluster of attractive women and spews out a string of jokes that he has memorized for the occasion. Then he approaches various women throughout the night, sometimes making flirtatious, suggestive comments. His silly, drunken behavior doesn't get him any dates. The following day, he's embarrassed and ashamed.

THE DIAGNOSTIC AND STATISTICAL MANUAL-5 (DSM-5)

Every so many years, groups of mental health professionals provide research and clinical experience in order to develop a list of emotional disorders. They publish their findings in a manual referred to as the *DSM*. Currently, the field is using the fifth edition. The diagnoses allow professionals to communicate with a common language. However, the formal role of diagnoses has its detractors. Many professionals believe it's more useful to focus on symptoms as opposed to specific disorders. For your information, the *DSM-5* currently lists the following major categories of anxiety disorders:

- Generalized anxiety disorder (GAD)
- Social phobia
- Panic disorder
- Agoraphobia
- Specific phobias
- Separation anxiety disorder
- Selective mutism
- Anxiety disorder due to another medical condition

The previous few editions of *DSM* categorized obsessive compulsive disorder (OCD) and post-traumatic stress disorder (PTSD) as anxiety disorders. No longer. Today, OCD has its own section, Obsessive Compulsive Related Disorders, and PTSD is categorized as a Trauma-and Stressor-Related Disorder. The controversies surrounding these changes are complex. And in most people with emotional problems, there are almost always overlapping symptoms. In other words, someone with anxiety is likely to have at least a few symptoms in one diagnostic category and a few others in a different category.

Maurice has social anxiety. Drug and alcohol abuse often accompany social phobia because people with social phobia feel desperate to quell their anxious feelings. And drugs and alcohol offer a quick fix. Unfortunately, that fix often causes additional embarrassment and may lead to an addiction.

Beyond everyday anxiety

Of course, everyone feels a little panicked from time to time. People often say they feel panicked about an upcoming deadline, an impending presentation, or planning for a party. You're likely to hear the term used to describe concerns about rather mundane events such as these.

But people who suffer with *panic* are talking about entirely different phenomena. They have periods of stunningly intense fear and anxiety. If you've never had a panic attack, trust us, you don't want one. The attacks usually last about ten minutes, and many people who have them fully believe that they will die during the attack. Not exactly the best ten minutes of their lives. Panic attacks normally include a range of robust, attention-grabbing symptoms, such as

>> An irregular, rapid, or pounding heartbeat

>> Perspiring

>> A sense of choking, suffocation, or shortness of breath

>> Vertigo or lightheadedness

>> Pain or other discomfort in the chest

>> A feeling that events are unreal or a sense of detachment

>> Numbness or tingling

>> Hot or cold flashes

>> A fear of impending death, though without basis in fact

>> Stomach nausea or upset

>> Thoughts of going insane or completely losing control

Panic attacks begin with an event that triggers some kind of sensation, such as physical exertion or normal variations in physiological reactions. This triggering event induces physiological responses, such as increased levels of adrenaline. No problem so far.

But the otherwise normal process goes awry at the next step — when the person who suffers from panic attacks misinterprets the meaning of the physical symptoms. Rather than viewing the physical symptoms as normal, the person with panic disorder sees them as a signal that something dangerous is happening, such as a heart attack or stroke. That interpretation causes escalating fear and thus more physical arousal. Fortunately, the body can sustain such heightened physical responses only for a while, so it eventually calms down.

Professionals say that in order to have a formal diagnosis of panic disorder, panic attacks must occur more than once. People with panic disorder worry about when the next panic attack will come and whether they'll lose control. They often start changing their lives by avoiding certain places or activities.

The good news: Many people have a single panic attack and never have another one. So, don't panic if you have a panic attack. Maria's story is a good example of a one-time panic attack.

> **Maria** resolves to lose 20 pounds by exercising and watching what she eats. On her third visit to the gym, she sets the treadmill to a level six with a steep incline. Almost immediately, her heart rate accelerates. Alarmed, she decreases the level to three. She starts taking rapid, shallow breaths but feels she can't get enough air. Sweating profusely and feeling nauseous, she stops the machine and staggers to the locker room. She sits down; the symptoms intensify, and her chest tightens. She wants to scream but can't get enough air. She's sure that she'll pass out and hopes someone will find her before she dies of a heart attack. She hears someone and weakly calls for help. An ambulance whisks her to a nearby emergency room.
>
> At the ER, Maria's symptoms subside, and the doctor explains the results of her examination. He says that she has apparently experienced a panic attack and inquires about what may have set it off. She answers that she was exercising because of concerns about her weight and health.
>
> "Ah, that explains it," the doctor reassures. "Your concerns about health made you hypersensitive to any bodily symptom. When your heart rate naturally increased on the treadmill, you became alarmed. That fear caused your body to produce more adrenaline, which in turn created more symptoms. The more symptoms you had, the more your fear and adrenaline increased. Knowing how this works may help you; hopefully, in the future, your body's normal physical variations won't frighten you. Your heart's in great shape. Go back to exercising.
>
> "Also, you might try some simple relaxation techniques; I'll have the nurse come in and tell you about those. I have every reason to believe that you won't have another episode like this one."
>
> Maria had one panic attack and may never experience another one. If she believes the doctor and takes his advice, the next time her heart races, she probably won't get so scared. She may decide to see how things go before seeking treatment for her problem. However, if she has a recurrence, treatment works pretty well for this issue.

HELP! I'M DYING!

Panic attack symptoms, such as chest pain, shortness of breath, nausea, and intense fear, often mimic heart attacks. Alarmed, those who experience these terrifying episodes take off in the direction of the nearest emergency room. Then, after numerous tests come back negative, overworked doctors tell the victim of a panic attack in so many words that "It's all in your head." Many patients with panic attacks doubt the judgment of the physician and strongly suspect that something important was missed or wasn't found.

The next time an attack occurs, panic attack victims are likely to return to the ER for another opinion. Even a second or third visit may not convince those with panic attacks that the feeling wasn't caused by a heart problem. The repeat visits frustrate people with panic attacks as well as ER staff. However, a simple 20- or 30-minute psychological intervention in the emergency room decreases the repeat visits dramatically. The intervention is pretty simple — just providing education about what the disorder is all about and describing a few deep relaxation techniques to try when panic hits.

Panic's companion

Approximately half of those who suffer from panic attacks have an accompanying problem: *agoraphobia.* Unlike most fears or phobias, this anxiety problem usually begins in adulthood. Individuals with agoraphobia symptoms live in terror of being trapped and unable to escape. They desperately avoid situations from which they can't readily escape, and they also fear places where help may not be readily forthcoming should they need it.

The agoraphobic may start with one fear, such as being in a crowd, but in many cases the feared situations multiply to the point that the person fears even leaving home. As agoraphobia teams up with panic, the double-barreled fears of not getting help and of feeling entombed with no way out can lead to paralyzing isolation.

You or someone you love may struggle with agoraphobia if

>> You worry about being somewhere where you can't get out or can't get help in case something bad happens, like a panic attack.

>> You tremble over everyday things like leaving home, being in large groups of people, or traveling.

>> Because of your anxiety, you avoid the places that you fear so much that it takes over your life, and you become a prisoner of your fear.

You may have concerns about feeling trapped or have anxiety about crowds and leaving home. Many people do. But if your life goes on without major changes or constraints, you're probably not agoraphobic.

For example, imagine that you quake at the thought of entering large sports stadiums. You see images of crowds pushing and shoving, causing you to fall over the railing, landing below, only to be trampled by the mob as you cry out. You may be able to live an entire blissful life avoiding sports stadiums. On the other hand, if you love watching live sports events, or you just got a job as a sports reporter, this fear could be *really bad.*

Luciana's story, which follows, demonstrates the overwhelming anxiety that often traps agoraphobics.

> **Luciana** celebrates her 40th birthday without having experienced significant emotional problems. She has gone through the usual bumps in the road of life like losing a parent, her child having a learning disability, and a divorce ten years earlier. She prides herself in coping with whatever cards life deals her.
>
> Lately, she feels stressed when shopping at the mall on weekends because of the crowds. She finds a parking spot at the end of a row. As she enters the mall, her sweaty hands leave a smudge on the revolving glass door. She feels as though the crowd of shoppers is crushing in on her, and she feels trapped. She worries she might faint, and no one would be there to help her. She's so scared that she flees the store.
>
> Over the next few months, her fears spread. Although they started at the mall, fear and anxiety now overwhelm her in crowded grocery stores as well. Later, simply driving in traffic scares her. Luciana suffers from agoraphobia. More and more she feels like staying in her house.

Many times, panic, agoraphobia, and anxiety strike people who are otherwise devoid of serious, deep-seated emotional problems. So, if you suffer from anxiety, it doesn't necessarily mean you'll need years of psychotherapy. You may not like the anxiety, but you don't have to think you're nuts!

Phobias: Spiders, snakes, airplanes, and other scary things

Many fears appear to be hard-wired into the human brain. Cave men and women had good reasons to fear snakes, strangers, heights, darkness, open spaces, and the sight of blood — snakes could be poisonous, strangers could be enemies, a person could fall from a height, darkness could harbor unknown hazards, open spaces could leave a primitive tribe vulnerable to attack from all sides, and the sight of blood could signal a crisis, even potential death. Fear fuels caution and avoidance of harm. Those with these fears had a better chance of survival than the naively brave.

That's why many of the most common fears today reflect the dangers of the world thousands of years ago. Even today, it makes sense to cautiously identify a spider before you pick it up. However, sometimes fears rise to a disabling level. You may have a *phobia* if

>> You have an exaggerated fear of a specific situation or object.

>> When you're in a fearful situation, you experience excessive anxiety immediately. Your anxiety *may* include sweating, rapid heartbeat, a desire to flee, tightness in the chest or throat, or images of something awful happening.

>> You know the fear is unreasonable. However, kids with specific phobias don't always know that their phobia is unreasonable. For example, they may really think that *all* dogs bite. (See Chapter 19 for more on phobias in children.)

>> You avoid your feared object or situation as much as you possibly can.

>> Because your fear is so intense, you go so far as to change your day-to-day behavior at work, at home, or in relationships. Thus, your fear inconveniences you and perhaps others, and it restricts your life.

REMEMBER

Almost two-thirds of people fear one thing or another. For the most part, those fears don't significantly interfere with everyday life. For example, if you fear snakes but don't run into too many snakes, then your fear can't really be considered a phobia. However, if your snake fear makes it impossible for you to walk around in your neighborhood, go on a picnic, or enjoy other activities, then it may be a full-blown phobia.

The following description of Dylan's life is a prime picture of what someone with a specific phobia goes through.

> **Dylan** trudges up eight flights of stairs each morning to get to his office and tells everyone that he loves the exercise. When Dylan passes the elevators on the way to the stairwell, his heart pounds, and he feels a sense of doom. Dylan envisions being boxed inside the elevator — the doors slide shut, and there's no escape. In his mind, the elevator box rises on rusty cables, makes sudden jerks up and down, falls freely, and crashes into the basement.

Dylan has never experienced anything like his fantasy, nor has anyone he knows had this experience. Dylan has never liked elevators, but he didn't start avoiding them until the past few years. It seems that the longer he stays away from riding them, the stronger his fear grows. He used to feel okay on escalators, but now he finds himself avoiding those as well. Several weeks ago at the airport, he had no alternative but to take the escalator. He managed to get on but became so frightened that he had to sit down for a while after he reached the second floor.

One afternoon, Dylan rushed down the stairs after work, running late for an appointment. He slipped and fell, breaking his leg. Now in a cast, Dylan faces the challenge of his life — with a broken leg, he now must take the elevator to get to his office. Dylan has a phobia.

Dylan's story illustrates how a phobia often starts out small and spreads. Such phobias gradually grow and affect one's life increasingly over time.

Rare symptoms of anxiety in adults

A couple of anxiety symptoms that usually occur in children sometimes follow into adulthood. As with other symptom clusters of anxiety, they often manifest themselves along with some degree of worry, panic, social fears, and so on. Two interesting though rare disorders include

>> **Separation anxiety disorder:** People who feel terrified that someone they love will be killed, kidnapped, injured, or die from an illness and as a result, refuse to be separated from their loved one. When separated, they often feel panic, extreme distress, and despair. The technical diagnosis is called *separation anxiety disorder.*

>> **Selective mutism:** Although this pattern usually begins in childhood, some adults are almost unable to speak in a variety of anxiety-arousing situations. They may neglect to say basics like "thank you" or "hello," not because of rudeness, but because of extreme fear. This form of anxiety can cause massive social and occupational limitations. This form of anxiety is technically known as *selective mutism.*

Anxiety symptoms can also be a direct consequence of certain medical conditions. Common conditions that can lead to significant anxious feelings include endocrine disorders; heart problems, especially arrhythmia; chronic obstructive pulmonary disease (COPD); and certain disorders of the brain.

How Anxiety Differs from Other Emotional Disorders

Anxious symptoms sometimes travel with other company. Thus, you may have anxiety along with other emotional disorders. In fact, about half of those with anxiety disorders develop depression, especially if their anxiety goes untreated. Recognizing the difference between anxiety and other emotional problems is important because the treatments differ somewhat.

>> **Obsessive compulsive disorder:** A person with OCD may exhibit behaviors that include an obsession, a compulsion, or both. *Obsessions* are unwelcome, disturbing, and repetitive images, impulses, or thoughts that jump into the mind. Most people who have OCD know that their obsessions are not entirely realistic but can't seem to stop believing them. Compulsions are repetitive actions or mental strategies carried out to temporarily reduce anxiety or

distress. Sometimes, an obsessive thought causes the anxiety; at other times, the anxiety relates to some feared event or situation that triggers the compulsion.

OCD used to be considered an anxiety disorder. Although OCD certainly involves some anxiety, recent research indicates that it affects different parts of the brain than anxiety. OCD also entails problems with impulsivity that are less common in anxiety.

>> **Post-traumatic stress disorder (PTSD):** You may have PTSD if you experience or witness an event that you perceive as life-threatening, causing serious injury, or sexual violence, and you feel terror, horror, or helplessness. You may also get PTSD from being a first responder witnessing trauma or by being close to someone who has been traumatized. You relive the event through flashbacks or memories. You try to avoid reminders of the event. Your thoughts and moods may be bleak, irritable, and easily triggered.

PTSD used to be considered an anxiety disorder. It was moved into a category of trauma disorders. Although PTSD does usually include anxiety symptoms, it also frequently is accompanied by anger, self-destructive behavior, and feelings of unreality.

>> **Depression:** Depression can feel like life in slow motion. You lose interest in activities that used to bring you pleasure. You feel sad. Most likely, you feel tired, and you sleep fitfully. Your appetite may wane, and your sex drive may droop. Similar to anxiety, you may find it difficult to concentrate or plan ahead. But unlike anxiety, depression saps your drive and motivation. For more information, see our book *Depression For Dummies* (Wiley).

>> **Bipolar disorder:** If you have bipolar disorder, you seesaw between ups and downs. At times, you feel that you're on top of the world. You believe your ideas are unusually important and need little sleep for days at a time. You may feel more special than other people. You may invest in risky schemes, shop recklessly, engage in sexual escapades, or lose your good judgment in other ways. You may start working frantically on important projects or find ideas streaming through your mind. Then suddenly you crash and burn. Your mood turns sour and depression sets in. (Check out *Bipolar Disorder For Dummies* by Candida Fink, MD, and Joe Kraynak [Wiley] for more about this disorder.)

>> **Psychosis:** Not only may psychosis make you feel anxious, but the symptoms also profoundly disrupt your life. Psychosis weaves hallucinations into everyday life. For example, some people hear voices talking to them or see shadowy figures when no one is around. Delusions, another feature of psychosis, also distort reality. Common psychotic delusions include believing that the CIA or aliens are tracking your whereabouts. Other delusions involve

grandiose, exaggerated beliefs, such as thinking you're Jesus Christ or that you have a special mission to save the world.

REMEMBER

If you think you hear the phone ringing when you're drying your hair or in the shower, only to discover that it wasn't, you're not psychotic. Most people occasionally hear or see trivial things that aren't there. Psychosis becomes a concern only when these perceptions seriously depart from reality. Fortunately, anxiety disorders don't lead to psychosis.

>> **Substance abuse:** When people develop a dependency on drugs or alcohol, withdrawal may create serious anxiety. The symptoms of drug or alcohol withdrawal include tremors, disrupted sleep, sweating, increased heartbeat, agitation, and tension. However, if these symptoms only come on in response to a recent cessation of substance use, they don't constitute an anxiety disorder.

WARNING

Those with anxiety disorders sometimes abuse substances in a misguided attempt to control their anxiety. If you think you have an anxiety disorder, be very careful about your use of drugs or alcohol. Talk to your doctor if you have concerns.

Chapter **3**

Investigating the Brain and Biology

Most people with anxiety describe uncomfortable physical symptoms that go along with their worries. They may experience heart palpitations, nausea, dizziness, sweats, or muscle tension. Those symptoms are evidence that anxiety is truly a disorder of both the mind and the body.

In this chapter, we review some of the biological roots of anxiety, as well as the consequences of chronic stress on health. Then we tell you about medications or food that can actually make you feel anxious. Finally, we discuss how some illnesses can cause or mimic anxiety.

Examining the Anxious Brain

The brain takes in information about the world through sight, taste, smell, sound, and touch. Constantly scanning the world for meaning, the brain integrates information from the past with the present and plans what actions to take. For most people, most of the time, the brain does a pretty good job. But for those with chronic anxiety, something goes awry.

Billions of nerve cells (*neurons*) reside in the brain. They're organized into a variety of complex structures or circuits. Some of these structures are particularly involved in producing feelings of anxiety, fear, and stress. These brain structures communicate with one another by sending chemical messengers, known as *neurotransmitters*, back and forth among them.

In the following sections, we explain how the brain interprets information and what role the brain's chemicals play in making you anxious.

How the brain's circuits connect

Think of the brain as having many interconnected circuits. One circuit involves both the *limbic system* and the *frontal lobes*. To keep it simple, the limbic system is a primitive region of the brain and is responsible for immediate reflexive responses to threat. The thalamus and the amygdala form part of the limbic system. The frontal lobes, which handle judgment and reasoning, respond more slowly and thoughtfully.

When the brain perceives something as being dangerous, it immediately registers in the brain's control center known as the thalamus. The thalamus rapidly sends a signal directly to the amygdala, which activates reflexive fear responses. Those responses prepare the body to fight or flee. The thalamus also delivers a warning signal through the frontal lobes. The frontal lobes, where rational thought occurs, take a little more time and use reason and logic to determine the veracity of the incoming threat. That's why when you perceive something as being scary, your body immediately responds with a rapid heartbeat, tension, and dread. If and when the rational frontal lobes figure out that the scary thing actually doesn't pose a significant threat, you calm down. That's the way the brain is supposed to work.

For example, around the Fourth of July you hear loud popping sounds. Your limbic system may initially interpret those as gunshots, but your frontal lobes take a few seconds longer and conclude that the sounds are likely to be firecrackers. However, dogs, who don't understand calendars or have well-developed frontal lobes, remain fearful.

In anxiety disorders, either the limbic system or the frontal lobes (or both) may fail to function properly. Thus, the limbic system may trigger fear responses too easily and too often, or the frontal lobes may fail to use logic to quell fears set off by the limbic system. When the brain signals danger, the body responds by getting ready for action. The next section explains the chemical aspects of fear.

Neurotransmitters

Neurotransmitters help nerve cells communicate feelings, fears, emotions, thoughts, and actions through an intricate orchestration. Four major neurotransmitter systems and some of their functions include

>> The *noradrenergic system,* which produces norepinephrine and epinephrine. It also stimulates organs required in the fight-or-flight response (see the following section).

>> The *cholinergic system,* which activates the noradrenergic neurotransmitters and facilitates formation of memories.

>> The *dopaminergic system,* which is involved in movement and is also related to feelings of pleasure and reward. Dopamine disruptions cause problems with attention, motivation, and alertness, and appear to be quite important in the development of fear responses.

>> The *serotonergic system,* which is related to moods, anxiety, and aggression.

STRESS AND VULNERABILITY TO INFECTION

A significant body of research spanning decades of work has linked stress and susceptibility to infections. This finding appears to be due to reductions in immune response and increased inflammation in highly stressed individuals. A recent study reported in the *British Medical Journal* looked at large groups of people with stress disorders, their siblings, and a group of people without stress disorders from the general population of Sweden.

After following the subjects for over 25 years, researchers found that people with stress disorders were significantly more prone to infections, including life-threatening infections. The study controlled for economic factors, family background, prior medical history, and a host of other variables.

The study may have implications for new viral infections as they inevitably arise. People with high levels of stress may be more susceptible to becoming infected as well as have a more difficult time recovering than those with lower stress levels. Furthermore, some research suggests that people with high levels of stress may not benefit as much as others from vaccinations. Thus, managing stress and anxiety may improve important health outcomes. These findings may ultimately prove to be especially important during times of pandemics.

As these neurotransmitters pulse through your brain, the brain circuitry involved in fear and anxiety lights up. Your body then responds with a full-system alert known as the fight-or-flight response.

Preparing to Fight or Flee

When danger presents itself, you reflexively prepare to stand and fight or run like you've never run before. Your body mobilizes for peril in complex and fantastic ways. Figure 3-1 gives you the picture.

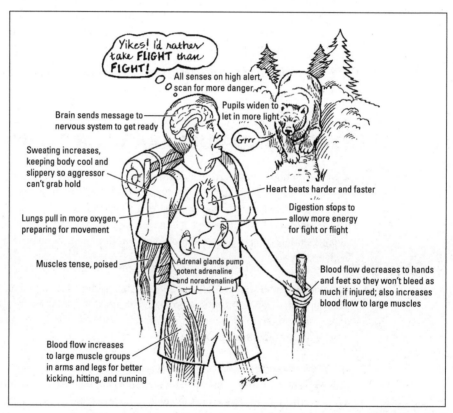

FIGURE 3-1: When presented with danger, your body prepares itself to flee or stand and fight.

Your body responds to threats by preparing for action in three different ways: physically, mentally, and behaviorally.

>> **Physically:** The brain sends signals through your nervous system to go on high alert. It tells the adrenal glands to rev up production of adrenaline and

noradrenaline. These hormones stimulate the body in various ways. Your heart pounds faster, and you start breathing more rapidly, sending increased oxygen to your lungs while blood flows to the large muscles, preparing them to fight or flee from danger.

Digestion slows to preserve energy for meeting the challenge, and pupils dilate to improve vision. Blood flow decreases to hands and feet to minimize blood loss if injured and keep up the blood supply to the large muscles. Sweating increases to keep the body cool, and it makes you slippery so aggressors can't grab hold of you. All your muscles tense to spring into action.

>> **Mentally:** You automatically scan your surroundings intensely. Your attention focuses on the threat at hand. In fact, you can't attend to much of anything else.

>> **Behaviorally:** You're now ready to run or fight. You need that preparation in the face of danger. When you have to take on a bear, a lion, or a warrior, you'd better have all your resources on high alert.

Granted, in today's world, you're not very likely to encounter lions and bears. Unfortunately, your body reacts too easily with the same preparation to fight traffic, meet deadlines, speak in public, and cope with other everyday worries.

When human beings have nothing to fight or run from, all that energy has to be released in other ways. So, you may feel the urge to fidget by moving your feet and hands. You may feel like jumping out of your skin. Or, you may impulsively rant or rave with those around you.

WARNING

Most experts believe that experiencing these physical effects of anxiety on a frequent, chronic basis doesn't do you any good. Various studies have suggested that chronic anxiety and stress contribute to a variety of physical problems, such as abnormal heart rhythms, high blood pressure, irritable bowel syndrome, asthma, ulcers, stomach upset, acid reflux, chronic muscle spasms, tremors, chronic back pain, tension headaches, a depressed immune system, and even hair loss. Figure 3-2 illustrates the toll of chronic anxiety on the body.

Before you get too anxious about your anxiety, please realize that chronic anxiety contributes to many of these problems, but we don't know for sure that it's a major cause of all of them. Nevertheless, enough studies have suggested that anxiety or stress can make these disorders worse to warrant taking chronic anxiety seriously. In other words, be concerned, but don't panic.

TECHNICAL STUFF

When people perceive danger, their most common response is to fight or flee. However, sometimes there is another reaction — freezing. This response is common in animals but less understood in humans. The well-known phrase "like a deer caught in the headlights" is an example of a freeze response. During this state, heart rate actually decreases, and the body becomes immobilized. Usually, this state is brief and can immediately change to fight or flight. This phenomenon explains why some people freeze during an emergency or find themselves unable to respond in a threatening situation. However, not as much is known about the human freeze response, and more research is needed to explain the nuances of why and when this occurs.

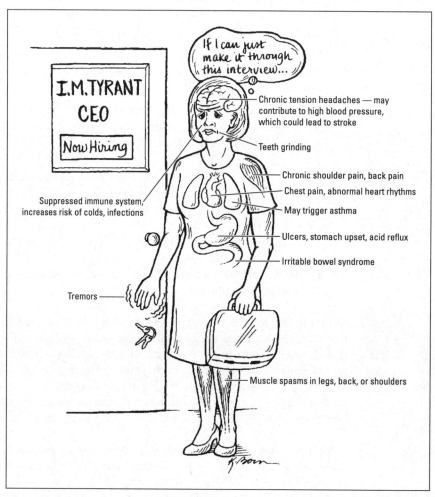

FIGURE 3-2:
The chronic effects of anxiety.

ANXIETY AND DIABETES

People with diabetes are at higher risk for developing anxiety. And people with anxiety are at higher risk of developing type 2 diabetes. Anxiety triggers the release of hormones that increase the levels of glucose (sugar) in the bloodstream. That release of excess sugar contributes to the development and/or exacerbation of diabetes.

In the other direction, diabetes can lead to anxiety because of perceived loss of health. Diabetes necessitates significant changes in lifestyle and increased attention and time for dealing with the control of blood sugar levels. Most people with diabetes also are well aware of complications such as increased risks for heart disease, glaucoma, neuropathy, and more.

The interaction of diabetes making stress worse and stress making diabetes harder to control calls for addressing the role of anxiety and stress in the improved management of diabetes. People with diabetes benefit from learning stress and anxiety management skills. In fact, glucose levels in people with diabetes generally decrease when anxiety is well controlled. So, if you don't have diabetes, protect yourself by overcoming anxiety, and if you do have diabetes, know that anxiety management may help you control the disease.

Mimicking Anxiety: Drugs, Diet, and Diseases

As common as anxiety disorders are, believing that you're suffering from anxiety when you're not is all too easy. Prescription drugs may have a variety of side effects, some of which mimic a few of the symptoms of anxiety. Sometimes what you eat or drink can make you feel anxious. Various medical conditions also produce symptoms that imitate the signs of anxiety. We look at these anxiety imitators in the following sections.

Exploring anxiety-mimicking drugs

Medicines prescribed to treat common conditions, such as asthma, inflammation, and depression, often have side effects. Sometimes those side effects can resemble the symptoms of anxiety. We list a few of the most widely prescribed types of drugs and their anxiety-mimicking side effects in Table 3-1. These medications have many other side effects that we don't list here.

TABLE 3-1   **Angst in the Medicine Cabinet**

Drug Name or Category	Purpose	Anxiety-Like Side Effects
Angiotensin-converting enzyme (ACE) inhibitors	Reduce high blood pressure	Nervousness, dizziness, insomnia, headaches, nausea, vomiting, weakness
Corticosteroids	Treat arthritis, inflammation, and pain	Fatigue, anxiety, dizziness, nervousness, insomnia, nausea, vomiting, sweating, tremors, confusion, shortness of breath, irritability
Bronchodilators	Treatment of asthma	Trembling, nervousness, sweating, shakiness, feelings of panic
Benzodiazepines	Treat anxiety	Dizziness, headache, anxiety, tremors, stimulation, insomnia, nausea, diarrhea, irritability
Beta blockers	Reduce angina and high blood pressure, treat dysrhythmia	Dizziness, nausea, palpitations, insomnia, excessive sweating, disorientation
Novocaine	Still used by some dentists as a numbing agent, but newer agents are becoming more popular due to reduced side effects.	Rare side effects can include anxiety, irregular heart beat, and dizziness, which are especially troubling for patients who already have dentist-related anxiety.
Selective serotonin reuptake inhibitors (SSRIs)	Treatment of depression, anxiety, and bulimia	Headache, insomnia, anxiety, tremor, dizziness, nervousness, fatigue, poor concentration, agitation, nausea, diarrhea, decreased appetite, sweating, hot flashes, palpitations, twitching, impotence
Stimulant medications	Treatment of attention deficit disorder	Nervousness, rapid heartbeat, disturbed sleep, panic feelings
Thyroid replacement medications	Treatment of hypothyroidism	Hives, chest pain, irregular heartbeat, nervousness, shortness of breath

Interesting, isn't it? Even medications for the treatment of anxiety can produce anxiety-like side effects. Of course, most people don't experience such side effects with these medications, but they do occur. And many other prescribed drugs may have anxiety-like side effects. If you're taking one or more prescription drugs and feel anxious, check with your doctor.

REMEMBER

In addition, various over-the-counter medications sometimes have anxiety-mimicking side effects. These include antihistamines that can cause both drowsiness and insomnia as well as restlessness and rapid heartbeat. Decongestants can also cause rapid heartbeat as well as sweating, dizziness, and blurred vision. Also, many types of aspirin contain caffeine, which can produce symptoms of anxiety if consumed excessively. These medications can cause restlessness, heart palpitations, tension, shortness of breath, and irritability.

Ingesting calmness into your diet

Stress and anxiety often provoke people to binge on unhealthy foods and substances, which may lead to increased anxiety over the long run. In Chapter 11, we discuss foods that may help you calm your moods and alleviate your anxiety. Here, we tell you how to avoid foods or drinks that may worsen problems with anxiety.

TIP

Notice whether you have special sensitivities to certain types of food. Whenever you feel out of sorts or especially anxious for no particular reason, ask yourself what you've eaten in the past couple hours. Take notes for a few weeks. Although food sensitivities aren't generally a major cause of anxiety, some people have adverse reactions to certain foods, such as nuts, wheat, dairy, shellfish, or soy. If your notes say that's true for you, avoid these foods!

Alcohol may be very tempting to people with anxiety. Although alcohol may relax you in small quantities, too many anxious people try to self-medicate by imbibing. People with anxiety disorders easily become addicted to alcohol. Furthermore, in excess, alcohol can lead to a variety of anxiety-like symptoms. For example, after a night of heavy drinking, alcohol can leave you feeling more anxious because it clears the system quickly and the body craves more. That craving can lead to addiction over time. Even a couple of glasses of wine in the evening may help you sleep initially but disturb the quality of your sleep leading to fatigue in the morning. So, anxious people need to be cautious about their use of alcohol.

Caffeine can also spell trouble. Some people seem to thrive on triple espressos, but others find themselves up all night with the jitters. Caffeine lurks in most energy drinks as well as chocolate, so be careful if you're sensitive to the effects of caffeine.

WARNING

Speaking of energy drinks, these sometimes contain unusually large quantities of not only caffeine but also other stimulants. You'll see herbal stimulants such as taurine, guarana (loaded with caffeine), ginseng, and ginkgo biloba, among others. Reported adverse effects include nervousness, sleeplessness, abnormal heart rhythms, and seizures. If you have excessive anxiety, you don't want to be chugging down these concoctions.

Finally, lots of people get nervous after eating too much sugar. Watch kids at birthday parties or Halloween. Adults can have the same reaction. Furthermore, sugar is bad for your body in a variety of ways, such as spiking blood glucose levels and contributing to metabolic syndrome (a condition that often leads to high blood pressure and diabetes).

THE CHICKEN OR THE EGG: IRRITABLE BOWEL SYNDROME

Irritable bowel syndrome (IBS) is a common condition that involves a variety of related problems, usually including cramps or pain in the abdomen, diarrhea, and/or constipation. These occur in people with no known physical problems in their digestive systems. IBS negatively impacts the quality of life for the 10 to 20 percent of the population, mainly women, who suffer from it. For many years, doctors told most of their patients that irritable bowel syndrome was caused by stress, worry, and anxiety.

Genetic research has found various genes that may contribute to the emergence of IBS. However, the exact role that genes play in this disorder remains unclear. More research is needed.

There is no known cure for IBS, and treatments are targeted at symptoms. Various medications have been found to decrease some of the worst symptoms of IBS. In addition, psychotherapy that teaches relaxation techniques, biofeedback, and techniques for coping with anxiety and stress also improves IBS symptoms. So, at this point, no one really knows to what extent IBS is caused by physical causes, anxiety, or stress. It's more likely, however, that the mind and body interact in important ways that can't always be separated.

Investigating medical anxiety imposters

REMEMBER

More than a few types of diseases and medical conditions can create anxiety-like symptoms. That's why we strongly recommend that you visit your doctor, especially if you're experiencing significant anxiety for the first time. Your doctor can help you sort out whether you have a physical problem, a reaction to a medication, an emotionally based anxiety problem, or some combination of these. Table 3-2 lists just some of the medical conditions that produce anxiety symptoms.

Getting sick can cause anxiety, too. For example, if you receive a serious diagnosis of heart disease, cancer, or a chronic progressive disorder, you may develop anxiety about dealing with the consequences of what you've been told. The techniques we give you for dealing with anxiety throughout this book can help you manage this type of anxiety as well.

TABLE 3-2   **Medical Imposters**

Medical Condition	What It Is	Anxiety-Like Symptoms
Hypoglycemia	Low blood sugar; sometimes associated with other disorders or can occur by itself. A common complication of diabetes.	Confusion; irritability; trembling; sweating; rapid heartbeat; weakness; cold, clammy feeling
Hyperthyroidism	Excess amount of thyroid hormone. Various causes.	Nervousness, restlessness, sweating, fatigue, sleep disturbance, nausea, tremor, diarrhea
Other hormonal imbalances	Various conditions associated with fluctuations in hormone levels, such as premenstrual syndrome (PMS), menopause, or postpartum. Highly variable symptoms.	Tension, irritability, headaches, mood swings, compulsive behavior, fatigue, panic
Lupus	An autoimmune disease in which the patient's immune system attacks certain types of its own cells.	Anxiety, poor concentration, irritability, headaches, irregular heartbeat, impaired memory
Mitral valve prolapse	The mitral valve of the heart fails to close properly, allowing blood to flow back into the left atrium. Often confused with panic attacks in making the diagnosis.	Palpitations, shortness of breath, fatigue, chest pain, difficulty breathing
Heart disease (including arrhythmias and tachycardia)	Conditions that involve narrowed or blocked blood vessels, problems with muscle, valves, or rhythm	Shortness of breath, noticeable changes in rhythm or skipped beats, chest tightness or pain
Chronic lung conditions (e.g., COPD, asthma)	Irritation or damage to the lungs	Shortness of breath, tightness in the chest, feelings of not getting enough air, panic
Ménière's syndrome	An inner ear disorder that includes vertigo, loss of hearing, and ringing or other noises in the ear.	Vertigo that includes abnormal sensations associated with movement, dizziness, nausea, vomiting, and sweating

REMEMBER

When you notice new signs of anxiety, ponder what changes you've made in your life. Have you started a new medication? Is something unusually stressful going on? How is your health? Have you made major changes to your diet or exercise routines? Answers to these questions may give you clues as to what's causing your uptick in anxiety. But, it's never a bad idea to check out these symptoms with your primary healthcare provider to play it safe.

Chapter **4**

Clearing the Roadblocks to Change

W e're guessing if you're reading this book, you have some interest in the topic of anxiety, and maybe you or someone you care about struggles with the problem. You've come to the right place. This book gives you strategies that help people manage their anxiety. However, you should know that sometimes people start on the path to change with the best intentions, but as they move along, they suddenly encounter icy conditions, lose traction, spin their wheels, and slide off the road.

This chapter gives you ways to throw salt and sand on the ice and keep moving forward. First, we explain where anxiety comes from. When you understand the origins of anxiety, you can move from self-blame to self-acceptance, thus allowing yourself to direct your energy away from self-abuse and toward more productive activities. Next, we show you the other big barriers that block the way to change. We give you effective strategies to keep you safely on the road to overcoming anxiety. And finally, if you need some outside support, we give you suggestions on how to find professional help.

Digging Out the Roots of Anxiety

Anxiety doesn't come out of nowhere; rather, it typically stems from some combination of three major contributing factors. The primary villains underlying anxiety are

>> **Genetics:** Your biological inheritance

>> **Parenting:** The way that you were raised

>> **Anxiety-arousing experiences:** Unpredictable, upsetting, or scary events

Studies show that of those people who experience unanticipated traumas or unpredictable events, only a minority end up with severe anxiety. That's because anxiety stems from a combination of causes. So, someone with resilient genes may experience bad parenting and a series of anxiety-arousing events yet not suffer from serious bouts of anxiety later on. Someone else with less resilient genes could develop serious problems with anxiety. Furthermore, someone with anxiety-prone genes could have a great childhood and relatively few anxiety-arousing events and live a life without significant problems with anxiety.

REMEMBER

Everyone experiences some anxiety from time to time. It's only a problem when anxiety detracts from your overall well-being and quality of life.

Some people seem almost immune to developing anxiety, yet it's possible that life could deal them a blow that challenges their coping abilities in a way they couldn't expect. In the story that follows, Liz shows how someone can show resilience for many years yet be tipped over the edge by a series of noxious bullying from her peers.

> **Liz** manages to grow up in a drug war zone without developing terribly distressing symptoms. One night, bullets whiz through her bedroom window, and one pierces her abdomen. She shows surprising resilience during her recovery. Surely, she must have some robust anti-anxiety genes and perhaps some pretty good parents in order to successfully endure such an experience. However, during high school, she is targeted by bullies for her success in her high-school band. Her antagonists post photoshopped, embarrassing pictures of her on social media. She withdraws and starts avoiding friends. Her anxiety causes her to drop out of band, and her grades slip. She just doesn't have the resources to face this onslaught of stress.

Thus, as Liz's example illustrates, you can never know for certain the exact cause of anyone's anxiety. However, if you examine someone's childhood relationship with her parents, family history, and the various events in her life (such as relationships, accidents, disease, and so on), you can generally come up with good ideas as to why anxiety now causes problems. If you have anxiety, think about which of the causes of anxiety have contributed to your troubles.

What difference does it make where your anxiety comes from? Overcoming anxiety doesn't absolutely require knowledge of where it originated. The remedies change little whether you were born with anxiety or acquired it much later in your life.

The benefit of identifying the source of your anxiety lies in helping you realize anxiety isn't something you brought on yourself. Anxiety develops for a number of good, solid reasons, which we elaborate on in the following sections. The blame doesn't belong with the person who has anxiety.

REMEMBER

Guilt and self-blame only sap you of energy. They drain resources and keep your focus away from the effort required for challenging anxiety. By contrast, self-forgiveness and self-acceptance energize and even motivate your efforts (we cover these ideas later in the chapter).

It's in my genes!

If you suffer from excessive worries and tension, look at the rest of your family. Of those who have an anxiety disorder, typically about a quarter of their relatives suffer along with them. So, your Uncle Ralph may not struggle with anxiety, but Aunt Melinda or your sister Charlene just might.

Maybe you're able to make the argument that Uncle Ralph, Aunt Melinda, and your sister Charlene all had to live with Grandma, who'd make anyone anxious. In other words, they lived in an anxiety-inducing environment. Maybe it has nothing to do with their genes.

Various researchers have studied siblings and twins who live together to verify that genes do play an important role as to how people experience and cope with anxiety. As predicted, identical twins were far more similar to each other in terms of anxiety than fraternal twins or other siblings. But even if you're born with a genetic predisposition toward anxiety, other factors — such as environment, peers, and how your parents raised you — enter into the mix.

It's how I was raised!

Blaming parents for almost anything that ails you is easy. Parents usually do the best they can. Raising children poses a formidable task. So in most cases, parents don't deserve as much blame as they receive. However, they do hold responsibility for the way that you were brought up to the extent that it may have contributed to your woes.

Three parenting styles appear to foster anxiety in children:

>> **Over-protectors:** These parents shield their kids from every imaginable stress or harm. If their kids stumble, they swoop them up before they even hit

the ground. When their kids get upset, they fix the problem. Not surprisingly, their kids fail to find out how to tolerate fear, anxiety, or frustration.

>> **Over-controllers:** These parents micro-manage all their children's activities. They direct every detail from how they should play to what they should wear to how they solve arithmetic problems. They discourage independence and fertilize dependency and anxiety.

>> **Inconsistent responders:** The parents in this group provide their kids with erratic rules and limits. One day, they respond with understanding when their kids have trouble with their homework; the next day, they explode when their kids ask for help. These kids fail to discover the connection between their own efforts and a predictable outcome. Therefore, they feel that they have little control over what happens in life. It's no wonder that they feel anxious.

If you recognize your own parenting style in any of these descriptions and worry that your behavior may be affecting your child, flip to Chapter 20 to see how you can help your child overcome her anxiety.

TIP

During unpredictably tough times like a pandemic, parents may find themselves becoming overly controlling and/or overly protective. Parents also may seem inconsistent during a pandemic when the rules change because of changing health information. Those reactions are perfectly understandable. When life and death decisions are in play, an extra dose of caution is warranted. So, control and protect when it comes to critical threats to health. At the same time, try to find some decisions that your children can safely make on their own. It's important to give them a sense of independence and autonomy during such stressful times. You can do so by giving choices over clothing, types of masks, movies to watch, or family games to play.

It's the world's fault!

The world today moves at a faster pace than ever, and the workweek has gradually inched upward rather than the other way around. Modern life is filled with both complexity and danger. Perhaps that's why mental health workers see more people with anxiety-related problems than ever before. Four specific types of events can trigger a problem with anxiety, even in someone who has never suffered from it much before:

>> **Unanticipated threats:** Predictability and stability counteract anxiety; uncertainty and chaos fuel it. For example, **Calvin** works long hours to make a decent living. Nevertheless, he lives from paycheck to paycheck with little left for savings. A freak slip on an icy patch of sidewalk disables him for six weeks, and he has insufficient sick leave to cover his absence. He now worries obsessively over his ability to pay bills. Even when he returns to work, he worries more than ever about the next financial booby trap that awaits him.

>> **Escalating demands:** Having too much responsibility piled on your plate can make you anxious. **Jake** initially thinks that nothing is better than a promotion when his supervisor hands him a once-in-a-lifetime opportunity to direct the new high-risk research and development division at work. Jake never expected such a lofty position or the doubling of his salary this early in his career. Of course, new duties, expectations, and responsibilities come along for the ride. Jake now begins to fret and worry. What if he fails to meet the challenge? Anxiety starts taking over his life.

>> **Confidence killers:** Unexpected criticisms and rejections can certainly trigger anxiety. **Tricia** is on top of the world. She has a good job and feels ecstatic about her upcoming wedding. However, she is stunned when her fiancé backs out of the proposal. Now, she worries incessantly that something is wrong with her; perhaps she'll never have the life she envisioned for herself.

>> **Major threats:** No one ever wants to experience a horrifying or even life-threatening experience. Unfortunately, these bitter pills do happen. Horrific accidents, acts of terrorism, pandemics, natural disasters, battlefield injuries, and violence have occurred for centuries, and we suspect they always will. When they do, severe problems with anxiety often emerge. Thus, survivors of tsunamis often have residual anxiety for years because of the totally unexpected nature of the event.

Finding Self-Acceptance

Time and again, we see our worried, tense clients suffer from another needless source of pain. Their anxiety is bad enough, but they also pound on themselves *because* they have anxiety. Such self-abuse involves harsh, critical judgments. If you do this to yourself, we suggest that you try the following approach to self-acceptance.

TIP

Start by making a list of all the likely causes of your problems with anxiety. First, list any possible genetic contributions that you can think of in your relatives who may suffer from anxiety. Then, review how your parents may have either modeled anxiety or instilled it in you because of their over-controlling, over-protecting, or harsh, unpredictable parenting style. Then, review events in your world from the distant to recent past that were highly anxiety-arousing. Finally, after you list the likely culprits that led to your distress, ask yourself some questions like the ones that follow:

>> Did I ask for my anxiety?

>> Was there ever a time in my life that I actually wanted to feel anxious?

>> Am I primarily to blame for my worries?

- » What percentage of the blame can I realistically assign to myself as opposed to genes, parenting, and events, both old and new?
- » If a couple of friends of mine had troubles with anxiety, what would I say to them?
  - Would I think they were to blame?
  - Would I think as ill of them as I do myself?
- » Does thinking badly about myself help me to get over my anxiety?
- » If I decided to stop pummeling myself, would I have more energy for tackling my problems?

These questions can help you move toward self-acceptance and discover that having anxiety has nothing to do with your worth or value as a human being. Then, you just might lighten up on yourself a little. We recommend it highly. Mind you, people get down on themselves at times. But chronic, unrelenting self-abuse is another matter. If you find yourself completely unable to let go of self-abuse, you may want to seek professional help (see the related section at the end of this chapter). You can read more about self-acceptance in Chapter 8.

ANXIETY AMONG THE RICH AND FAMOUS

So many of our clients seem to think that they're the only people in the world who struggle with anxiety. But we let them know that many millions of Americans suffer from anxiety. Perhaps you won't feel quite so alone if you consider some of the famous people throughout history who've suffered from one or more of the various anxiety disorders discussed in this book.

Reportedly, Albert Einstein and Eleanor Roosevelt both suffered from fears of social situations. Further, Charles Darwin eventually became a virtual hermit because of his disabling agoraphobia (see Chapter 2). Robert Frost also battled anxiety.

Prince Harry went against royal tradition and admitted to having problems with mental health, including panic attacks. After losing his mother at the age of 12, he attempted to avoid suffering by failing to deal with stress and trauma in his life. Unfortunately, avoidance usually just makes anxiety worse, and it did for Prince Harry, until he sought professional help. Revealing his own struggles was a brave act, and he now works to encourage others to seek help for their emotional difficulties. Finally, a search on the internet shows you that hundreds of celebrities reputedly suffer from all kinds of severe problems with anxiety. Use a search engine and type in "famous people and anxiety." You'll be surprised by what you discover. But be aware that the internet is also full of foolish, incorrect information. So, view what you find with a critical eye.

Gavin's story illustrates how reviewing the causes of your anxiety, followed by asking yourself those important questions, can help you acquire self-acceptance.

Gavin has developed panic disorder gradually over the past couple of years. His attacks of feeling breathless, nauseous, dizzy, and thinking he's going crazy have increased recently. He feels shame that someone like him has this problem. When he starts having panic attacks at work, he seeks help. He tells his psychologist that a real man would never have this kind of problem. His psychologist helps Gavin to be more self-forgiving. He asks Gavin to write down the causes of his anxiety. He tells him to thoroughly review his life and come up with as many contributors to his anxiety as he can. Table 4-1 shows what Gavin comes up with.

By reviewing the causes of his anxiety and asking himself the questions listed earlier in this section, Gavin moves from self-abuse to self-acceptance. Now he's ready to work on overcoming his anxiety.

TABLE 4-1 **Gavin's Anxiety Causes**

Possible Genetic Influences	Parenting	Events: Old and New
My Aunt Mary hardly ever leaves her house. Maybe she has something like I do.	Well, my father had quite an unpredictable temper. I never knew when he'd blow.	When I was 6, we had a terrible car accident, and I spent three days in the hospital. I was very scared.
My mother is very high-strung.	My mother's moods bounced all over the place. I could never tell how she'd react when I asked her for something.	My middle school was in a terrible neighborhood. Gangs ruled. I had to look over my shoulder at every turn.
My cousin Margarite seems very shy. Maybe she has a lot of anxiety.		My first marriage ended when I caught my wife cheating. Even though I trust my new wife, I worry too much about her faithfulness.
My brother worries all the time. He seems totally stressed.		Two years ago, I was diagnosed with diabetes. I worry a lot about my health.

Having Second Thoughts about Change

Clearly, no one likes feeling anxious, tense, and nervous, and sometimes anxiety climbs to such heights that it overwhelms personal resources and the capacity to cope. Chronic, severe anxiety not infrequently serves as a prelude to serious depression. Obviously, anyone experiencing this torment would jump at the chance to do something about it.

With good intentions, people buy self-help books, attend workshops, and even seek therapy. They fully intend to make meaningful changes in their lives. But have you ever gone to a health club in January? It's packed with new, enthusiastic members. By mid-March, health clubs return to normal. Like so many New Year's resolutions, the initial burst of resolve too often fades. What happens to all that determination? Folks generally think they've simply lost their willpower. Actually, interfering thoughts creep into their minds and steal their motivation. They start to think that they don't have the time or the money or that they can get in shape later. Such thoughts seduce them into abandoning their goals.

Thoughts about abandoning your quest to overcome anxiety may disrupt your efforts at some point. If so, the first step involves identifying the thoughts that are streaming through your mind. The next step is to fight off these counterproductive thoughts; we give you strategies for doing just that in the following section. But first, here are our top ten excuses for staying stuck:

>> **Number 10:** Anxiety isn't really that big a problem for me. I thought it was when I bought this book, but my anxiety isn't as bad as some of the people I've been reading about. Maybe it's not that big a deal.

>> **Number 9:** If I try and fail, I'll make a fool of myself. My friends and family would think I was stupid to even try.

>> **Number 8:** My anxiety feels too overwhelming to tackle. I just don't know if I could handle the additional stress of even thinking about it.

>> **Number 7:** I'm afraid of trying and not getting anywhere. That would make me feel even worse than if I did nothing at all. I'd feel like a failure.

>> **Number 6:** Feelings can't really be controlled. You're just fooling yourself if you think otherwise. You feel the way you feel.

>> **Number 5:** I'll do something about my anxiety when I feel the motivation. Right now, I don't really feel like it. I'm sure the motivation will come; I just have to wait for it.

>> **Number 4:** Who would I be without my anxiety? That's just who I am. I'm an anxious person; it's just me.

>> **Number 3:** I don't believe I can really change. After all, I've been this way my entire life. Books like this one don't work anyway.

>> **Number 2:** I'm too busy to do anything about my anxiety. These activities look like they take time. I could never work it into my hectic schedule.

>> **And the number 1 reason people stay stuck:** I'm too anxious to do anything about my anxiety. Whenever I think about confronting my anxiety, it makes me even more anxious. Why bother?

Look over our preceding list several times. Mull over each excuse and circle any that seem familiar or reasonable to you. Agreeing with any of these will hinder your progress. Now, we have some ways for you to challenge these excuses, no matter how reasonable they may seem.

Deciding to Get the Show on the Road

If any of our top ten excuses for staying stuck (see the preceding section) resonate with you, then your decision to overcome anxiety is not stable. Those thoughts can sabotage your best intentions. Don't underestimate their power.

The next two sections show you a couple of strategies for helping you turn your intentions into actions.

REMEMBER

If you start losing your motivation or your belief in your ability to do something about your anxiety, come back to this section! It can help you get back on track.

Arguing with your arguments

TIP

Consider starting a notebook or keeping a file for carrying out various exercises in this book. Whether you use a notebook, your phone, or another device, divide a page into two columns. Label the left column "Excuses" and the right column "Arguments Against My Excuses." Under "Excuses" write each of the top ten excuses (see the earlier section "Having Second Thoughts about Change") that apply to you. Then, as a way to come up with arguments against your excuses, ask yourself the following questions:

>> Does my excuse presume a catastrophe is coming?

>> Am I exaggerating the truth?

>> Can I find any evidence that would contradict my excuse?

>> Can I think of people to whom my excuse doesn't apply? And if it doesn't apply to them, why should it apply to me?

>> Am I trying to predict the future with negative thinking when no one can ever know the future?

Using those questions to guide your effort, jot down the best arguments you can for picking your excuses apart. The following example of Miguel shows how he attacked his most stubborn excuses for not changing.

Miguel suffers from anxiety and has resisted dealing with his problem for years. He lists his major excuses for not doing anything and uses the preceding questions to develop arguments against each of his excuses. Table 4-2 shows what he came up with for what he considered his most compelling excuses.

TABLE 4-2   **Miguel's Excuses versus Arguments Against His Excuses**

Excuse for Staying Stuck	Arguments Against My Excuse
If I try and fail, I'll make a fool of myself. My friends and family would think I was stupid to even try.	What do I mean by "making a fool of myself?" A true fool wouldn't even try. My family and friends would applaud any positive attempt I made, whether I succeed or not.
Feelings can't really be controlled. You're just fooling yourself if you think otherwise. You feel the way you feel.	Evidence tells me I've made other changes in my life. Many people go to therapy for some reason; surely it makes them feel better or there wouldn't be a zillion therapists in the world. My best friend overcame his anxiety, so why can't I?

Miguel discovered that arguing against his excuses finally gave him the courage to start making changes. You can do the same. Spend some time looking at your excuses that cause you to delay or put off working on your anxiety. Realize that working on your anxiety will pay off over time.

Taking baby steps

If you find that the idea of dealing with your anxiety is just too much to handle, you may be struggling with excuse number 8 for staying stuck (see the earlier section "Having Second Thoughts about Change"): "My anxiety feels too overwhelming to tackle. I just don't know if I could handle the additional stress of even thinking about it." In this case, it may help if you start by putting one foot in front of the other — take baby steps.

Stop dwelling on the entire task. For example, if you thought about all the steps that you'll take over the next five years, you'd be envisioning an incredible amount of walking. Hundreds, if not thousands, of miles await you. The mere thought of all those miles could stress you out.

You may, like many folks, wake up early in the morning on some days facing huge lists of things you need to do in the coming week. Ugh. A sense of defeat sets in, and you feel like staying in bed for the rest of the day. Dread replaces enthusiasm. If, instead, you clear your mind of the entire agenda and concentrate on only the first item on the list, your distress is likely to diminish, at least a little.

In order to take baby steps, it's a good idea to write down your overall, endpoint goal. For example, perhaps you eventually hope to be able to give an hour-long speech in front of a crowd without being overcome with fear, or maybe you want to be able to master your fear of heights by taking a tramway to the top of a mountain.

TIP

Sit down and chart out your ultimate goal, and then chart a goal that isn't quite so lofty to serve as a stepping stone — an intermediate goal. Then chart out the action that would be required of you to meet that goal. If your intermediate goal feels doable, you can start with it. If not, break it down further into smaller goals, even baby steps. It doesn't matter how small you make your first step. Anything that moves you just a little in the right direction can get you going and increase your confidence with one step at a time. Here's how Alaina put this plan into action.

> **Alaina** has a social phobia. She can't stand the idea of attending social functions. She feels that the moment that she walks into a group, all eyes focus on her, which sends her anxiety through the roof. She desperately wants to change. But the idea of attending large parties or company functions overwhelms her with terror. Look at Table 4-3 to see how Alaina broke the task down into baby steps.

TABLE 4-3 **Alaina's Baby Steps to Success**

Goals	Step-by-Step Breakdown of Actions
Ultimate goal	Going to a large party, staying the entire time, and talking with numerous people without fear.
Intermediate goal	Going to a small party, staying a little while, and talking to a couple people although feeling a little scared.
Small goal	Going to a work-related social hour, staying 30 minutes, and talking to at least one person in spite of some anxiety.
First baby step	Texting a friend, asking her to go to lunch, and talking about her struggles, in spite of anxiety.

> Alaina found that starting with texting a friend for advice over lunch helped get her moving. She repeated going to lunch and seeking advice with a few more of her friends. From there, she took the next step and went to a work social event for 30 minutes. She enjoyed herself so much that she continued going to events. After getting closer to friends and work colleagues, she found attending a large party easy.

TIP

Most people find that breaking tasks down into many small steps helps, especially for formidable goals. Make the steps easy at first, getting a bit harder with each success.

PERSEVERING THROUGH THE PEAKS AND VALLEYS

Many psychologists have conducted extensive research on how people make important changes, such as quitting smoking, losing weight, and overcoming emotional difficulties. They found that change isn't a straightforward process. It includes a number of stages:

- **Precontemplation:** In this stage, people haven't even given a thought to doing anything about their problem. They may deny having any difficulty at all. They're unconcerned about possible negative effects anxiety may exert on their health or day-to-day ability to function well.

- **Contemplation:** Here, people begin to think about tackling their problem. They have a glimmer of an idea that anxiety is getting in the way of their own happiness. But in this stage, it feels a little out of their reach to do anything about it.

- **Preparation:** In the preparation stage, people develop a plan for change. They gather their resources and make resolutions. They may read books like this one, talk to friends about their problems, and possibly check out getting a referral to a mental health professional.

- **Action:** The real work begins, and the plan goes into action. Whether it's through support groups, individual therapy, or self-help, those in the action phase begin doing something active about their anxiety. They remain in this stage until goals are mostly met.

- **Maintenance:** Now is the time to hold one's ground. People must hang tough to prevent sliding back. During this phase, one wants to develop a plan for dealing with both expected and unexpected problematic events.

- **Termination:** The change has become habit, so much so that relapse is less likely, and further work isn't particularly necessary. Not exactly everyone reaches the full stage of termination. Most people continue to struggle from time to time. That's normal and rather expected.

These stages look like a straight line from precontemplation to termination, but what these psychologists found is that people bounce around the stages in various ways. They may go from contemplation to action without having made adequate preparation. Others may reach the maintenance stage and give up on their efforts, slipping back to the precontemplation stage.

Many successful changers bounce back and forth in these stages a number of times before finally achieving their goals. So, don't get discouraged if that happens to you. Keep your goal in mind, and restart your efforts if you slip. Yep. Try, try, and try again.

Watching Worries Come and Go

Sometimes anxiety feels like it will never go away. Believing that you have no control over it and that stress invades your every waking moment is easy. This section helps you to realize that anxiety actually has an ebb and flow. We show you how taking a few minutes to write down your feelings each day may discharge a little of your anxiety and possibly improve your health. We also help you understand that progress, like anxiety, ebbs and flows.

Following your fears

One of the best early steps that you can take to manage anxiety is to simply follow it every day in a couple of different ways. Why would you want to do that? After all, you already know full well that you're anxious. Watching your worries is a good idea because it starts the process of change. You discover important patterns, triggers, and insights into your anxiety.

Observing anxiety fulfills several useful functions. First, monitoring forces you to be aware of your emotions. Avoiding and running away from troubling emotions only causes them to escalate. Second, you'll see that your anxiety goes up and down throughout the day — which isn't quite as upsetting as thinking it rules every moment of your life. And, you're likely to discover that recording your ratings can help you take charge and feel more in control of what's going on inside of you. Finally, keeping track helps you see how you're progressing in your efforts to quell your distress.

TIP

Track your anxiety on your phone or in a notebook for a few weeks. Notice patterns or differences in intensity. Fill out your chart at the same time each day. On a scale of one to ten, ten being total panic and one being complete calm, rate the level of anxiety you experience around the same time in the morning, then again in the afternoon, and later in the evening. Virginia's story shows you how tracking anxiety can be helpful.

> **Virginia** complains to her friends that she's the most nervous person on the planet and that she's close to a nervous breakdown. Recently, her father had heart surgery, and her husband lost his job. Virginia feels completely out of control and says that her anxiety never stops. When her counselor suggests that she start tracking her anxiety, she tells him, "You've got to be kidding. I don't need to do that. I can tell you right now that I'm anxious all the time. There's no letup." He urges her to go ahead and try anyway. Table 4-4 shows what Virginia comes up with in her first week of tracking.

TABLE 4-4   **Virginia's Day-by-Day Anxiety Levels**

Day	Morning	Afternoon	Evening	Daily Average
Sunday	4	6	8	**6**
Monday	6	7	9	**7.3**
Tuesday	5	6	6	**5.7**
Wednesday	4	5	7	**5.3**
Thursday	3	8	8	**6.3**
Friday	5	9	9	**7.7**
Saturday	3	5	5	**4.3**
Average	**4.3**	**6.6**	**7.4**	**6.1**

Virginia discovers a few things. First, she notices that her anxiety is routinely less intense in the morning. It escalates in the afternoon and peaks in the evenings. With only one week's record, she can't discern whether her anxiety level is decreasing, increasing, or remaining stable. However, she notices feeling a little better simply because she feels like she's starting to take charge of her problem. She also realizes that some days are better than others and that her anxiety varies rather than constantly overwhelming her.

THE POWER OF POSITIVE PSYCHOLOGY

The field of psychology focused on negative emotions for most of the 20th century. Psychologists studied depression, anxiety, schizophrenia, behavior disorders, and a slew of other maladies. Only recently has the field looked at the pluses of positive emotions, the characteristics of happy people, and the components of well-being. People who feel grateful usually say they feel happier as well.

One study assigned people to three groups. The first group wrote only about the hassles of everyday life. The researchers asked the second group to write about emotionally neutral events. The third group journaled about experiences that they were grateful for. All the groups performed this task merely once a week for ten weeks. At the end of the experiment, the group that wrote about gratitude exercised more, had fewer physical complaints, and felt more optimistic than those in the other two groups. That such an easy, simple task could be so beneficial is surprising.

Later studies have found that journaling helps decrease anxiety associated with multiple sclerosis, as well as other health conditions. Furthermore, it decreases stress related to school pressures and everyday anxiety.

Writing about your worries

Millions of people keep a diary at some point in their lives. Some develop daily writing as a lifelong habit. Keeping a journal of life's emotionally significant events has surprising benefits:

>> Journal writing appears to decrease the number of visits people make to the doctor for physical complaints.

>> Writing increases the production of T cells that are beneficial to the immune system.

>> Keeping a journal about emotional events improved the grades of a group of college students compared to those who wrote about trivial matters.

>> Recently, unemployed workers who wrote about the trauma of losing their jobs found new employment more quickly than those who did not.

Throwing out the rule book

Journal writing doesn't have rules. You can write about anything, anywhere, anytime. However, if you want the full benefits of writing in a journal, we encourage you to write about feelings and the emotionally important events of your life. Write about anything that troubles you during the day and/or past difficulties. Spend a little time on it.

TIP

Most smartphones allow you to dictate your thoughts rather than type them in. That's pretty great if you don't like tapping on a small keyboard. Like a journal, save your musings in a file and review them from time to time.

WARNING

Writing about past traumas may bring considerable relief. However, if you find that the task floods you with overwhelming grief or anxiety, you'll probably find it helpful to seek professional assistance.

Counting your blessings: An antidote for anxiety

Writing about your distressing feelings makes a great start. However, if you'd like more bang for your buck, take a few extra minutes and write about what you feel grateful for each day. Why? Because positive emotions help counteract negative emotions. Writing about your boons and blessings improves mood, increases optimism, and may benefit your health.

At first blush, you may think that you have little to be grateful for. Anxiety can so easily cloud vision. Did your mother ever urge you to clean your plate because of the "starving kids in China"? As much as we think that pushing kids to eat is a bad idea, her notion to consider those less fortunate has value. Take some time to ponder the positive events and people in your life.

>> **Kindnesses:** Think about those who have extended kindness to you.

>> **Education:** Obviously, you can read; that's a blessing compared to the millions in the world with no chance for an education.

>> **Nourishment:** You probably aren't starving to death, whereas (as your mother may have noted) millions are.

>> **Home:** Do you live in a cardboard box or do you have a roof over your head?

>> **Pleasure:** Can you smell flowers, hear birds sing, or touch the soft fur of a pet?

Sources of possible gratitude abound — freedom, health, companionship, and so on. Everyone has a different list. Start yours now.

TIP

The brain tends to focus on what's wrong or threatening in our lives. Noticing and actively appreciating what's right helps counteract that tendency and will make you feel better.

Getting Help from Others

If your problems with anxiety are significantly interfering with your life, you're probably going to want to work with a mental health professional in addition to reading this book. In the following two sections, we tell you what kind of treatment to ask for and give you a set of questions to ask a potential therapist before you begin treatment.

Seeking the right therapies

Mental health professionals offer a wide variety of treatments. We've thoroughly studied the research on what works for anxiety disorders so you don't have to. The best treatments for anxiety have been based on scientific knowledge about what anxiety is and how it works. Studies *consistently* show that treatments with this scientific foundation are particularly effective. Four treatments have shown efficacy over time:

>> **Cognitive therapy (CT)** focuses on teaching you new ways of *thinking*. People with anxiety often have distortions in the way they perceive events, and this

approach helps you correct those distortions. For example, an anxious client may be overestimating the risks involved with flying. A cognitive approach would help her discover that the risks are small enough to warrant tackling her fear.

>> **Metacognitive therapy (MCT)** goes beyond cognitive therapy and targets the way people think about their thinking. So, it isn't just concerned with distortions in thinking; rather, it also focuses on how upset one gets over disturbing thoughts. For example, an anxious person may overestimate the risk of being rejected. Cognitive therapy would help that person reassess that risk. MCT would help the person realize that much of the upset is about viewing the distorted thought itself as horrible instead of just a random thought.

>> **Behavior therapy (BT)** operates on the premise that changing the way you *act* or *behave* changes the way you feel about the things that happen in your life. Using the previous example of the woman with a fear of flying, a behavior therapist would likely help the woman go through a series of steps related to flying such as watching movies of flying, going to the airport, and eventually booking and taking a flight. Exposure therapy is a primary tool used by behavior therapists when treating anxiety related problems. (See Chapter 9 for more information.).

>> **Acceptance and commitment therapy (ACT)** guides clients to become more mindful of the present moment. Thoughts and emotions must be accepted rather than avoided. The very attempt to avoid thoughts and emotions makes them worse according to ACT. ACT also encourages people to identify their core values and live life accordingly.

TECHNICAL
STUFF

One other therapy you may hear about is called cognitive behavior therapy (CBT), which essentially represents a combination of CT and BT. We write about these specific types of therapies to inform our readers about what research has found to be successful. In general, all these approaches seem to work. Many of the techniques in each therapy are similar and overlap. That fact may explain why outcome studies have not demonstrated clear superiority for one of these approaches over the others.

TIP

Treatments that work share similar strategies. Therefore, we select some of the best elements from each type of therapy for dealing with common symptoms of anxiety, as seen in Part 2.

Seeking the right therapist

In addition to knowing the right therapy, you need to know whom to look for. Start by making sure that the therapist you seek is licensed to provide mental health services, whether as a counselor, psychiatrist, psychiatric nurse, psychologist, or social worker. Sources for finding one of these licensed practitioners include local professional associations (such as state psychology associations, state counselor associations, and so forth), your primary healthcare provider, your insurance company, or trusted friends and family who can recommend someone.

After you've found a professional who seems to fit the bill, be sure to ask the following questions:

>> What are your charges for services, and does my insurance cover them?

>> What are your hours?

>> How soon can you see me?

>> What is your experience in treating anxiety disorders?

>> What therapy approach do you take in treating anxiety?

>> Are you willing to collaborate with my doctor?

REMEMBER

You should feel comfortable talking with your therapist. After a few sessions, you should feel listened to and understood and sense that your therapist has legitimate empathy and concern for your well-being. Don't hesitate to inquire about the nature of your treatment plan — that plan should make sense to you. Most therapists take a few weeks getting to know you before they formulate an entire plan. If you're uncomfortable for any reason, by all means seek a second opinion from another therapist. Research shows that how you feel about the relationship with your therapist makes a big difference in how well the therapy goes.

2
Battling Anxiety

Recognize the difference between thoughts and feelings.

Figure out how to rethink anxious thoughts.

Dig into assumptions that make you anxious.

Learn to welcome anxious feelings.

Explore the pluses and minuses of medication.

Chapter **5**

Understanding Feelings

When you pass someone walking their dog, you might ask, "How are you doing today?" Most people will respond with something along the lines of "good," "fine," or "just great."

Is that really how they feel? Perhaps the person who said "fine" just found out he has stage four cancer. Or someone who said "good" recently won a million-dollar lottery. Fine or good hardly capture their true emotional experiences. People often have a discrepancy between the way they display emotion versus how they actually experience feelings. Sometimes that discrepancy is adaptive, whereas other times it's problematic.

In this chapter, we dig deep into emotions. We talk about emotional expression and emotional awareness. We show you how to uncover, understand, and appreciate your true emotions. Emotions are labels given to physiological sensations that occur in response to events.

The emotions actually experienced depend greatly on how you think about, interpret, and perceive events. In turn, how you think and feel influence how you behave or respond to what's happening. We describe how feeling, thinking, and behaving interact and give you strategies for tracking your upsetting emotions and the triggers that set them off. Keeping track of your emotions opens the door to relating to your feelings in a new, healthier way.

REMEMBER

Note, we use the terms emotions and feelings interchangeably. We could make nuanced distinctions between the two, but for simplicity's sake, we avoid that temptation.

What Do You Feel and Why?

Scientists who study emotions have recognized at least six primary emotions that occur across all human cultures. Other emotions such as anxiety or depression emerge from these primary emotions. You can probably think of hundreds of additional terms that describe other emotions (such as embarrassment, gloom, pride, contempt, shame, joy, dread, guilt, and so on). However, the primary six emotions include

>> Happiness

>> Sadness

>> Anger

>> Fear

>> Disgust

>> Surprise

Defining what an emotion is can be surprisingly difficult. Philosophers, psychologists, and scholars have debated for centuries about what an emotion is. There are as many definitions of emotions as there are flavors of gum. For the purpose of clarity, we like to think of emotions as a mixture of physical sensations and the labels we use to organize or describe them. These emotions or feelings are largely determined by thoughts and behaviors.

For example, an emotion may help you stay safe when you encounter a rattlesnake on a hike. You hear the rattle. The emotion of fear alerts you to the need for making a quick decision about the threat. Your body responds physiologically with adrenaline that creates fear, anxiety, and tension. You have thoughts that, "Oh, my God! It's a rattlesnake, and I may die!"

Then you have behaviors. Person A gasps, then slowly backs up. Person B screams and jumps. What then happens to persons A and B? The emotional response of fear can lead to a good or bad outcome.

WARNING

Just in case you didn't know, it's pretty much a bad idea to make sudden sounds and movements in response to a rattlesnake!

Emotions play a critical role in keeping you informed about what's going on in your world. Emotions capture your attention and focus your mind on what is important. In some cases, emotions lead you to productive behaviors; in other situations, they make things worse.

TIP

An emotion is a signal for alerting you to a significant event or memory. How you relate to the emotion determines whether your response is adaptive or misguided.

Feelings are sensational!

The human body is an exquisite tool that responds to millions of inputs throughout the day. The first signal of an emotional reaction is usually a physical feeling or body sensation, before the conscious mind is even aware that something is going on. The body reacts to threats (either real or perceived) with one or more of the following:

>> Rapid breathing

>> Shallow breathing

>> Shortness of breath

>> Tense muscles

>> Grinding teeth

>> Chest tightness

>> Stomach upset

>> Rapid pulse

>> Sweating

>> Fatigue

>> Dizziness

>> Retching

>> Blushing

These reactions generally occur suddenly, without warning. Pay attention to them when they pop up. They signal you that various emotions may be in play. Study those feelings and notice the context they're occurring in. You're likely to be able to come up with a label that describes the emotion that you are feeling (for example, anxiety, fear, distress).

WARNING

The physiological responses in the preceding list indicate emotions when they're relatively brief and happen during certain types of events (such as snakes, gunshots, and final exams). However, if you experience them chronically or not in the presence of an apparently stressful event, you should get checked out by a primary care provider. Once you have verified that you don't have a health condition, these physiological reactions may indicate excessive stress or anxiety.

Feelings tell you what to do

Feelings drive much of your behavior. Sometimes, without even thinking, your body has a sensation, and your actions follow. Here are a few examples to clarify this point:

>> When your body feels afraid, you try to leave or evade the situation.

>> When you feel sad, you withdraw from people and events.

>> When you feel happy, you approach people.

>> When you feel angry, you may complain, yell, or slam something.

>> When you're anxious, you try to avoid taking chances.

The emotions that emerge from your body push you to action or inaction. However, it's the way you think about, perceive, or interpret your feelings that is particularly influential in determining how you handle your feelings. (See Chapter 8 for information about emotions and behaviors.)

Feelings often arise from your thoughts

Thoughts powerfully influence your emotions. At the same time, your feelings also influence your thoughts. In order to battle anxiety, you need to be aware of both your thoughts and feelings.

The following true story from our lives illustrates how profoundly thoughts influence the way people feel.

A few years ago, we took a cruise to reward ourselves for completing a major project. One evening, we sat on deck chairs enjoying a fabulous sunset: Brilliant red and orange clouds melted into the deep blue sea. The wind picked up ever so slightly, and the ship rolled gently. We sat relaxed, quietly enjoying the scene and the cradle-like motion. We reflected that in our lifetime, we had rarely felt so at peace.

The captain's weather announcement interrupted our tranquil state of mind. Apologizing for the inconvenience, he informed us that because of a hurricane, he would have to steer a slightly different course, and we may feel some choppy seas. Still, he assured us that the storm presented no threat.

The breeze suddenly felt chilling. The clouds, so spectacular before, appeared ominous. The gentle roll that had relaxed us now generated nervousness. Yet nothing about the sky or the sea had changed from moments earlier.

Our thoughts jerked us from blissful relaxation to mounting anxiety. We pulled our jackets tighter and commented that the weather looked nasty, and perhaps we'd be better off inside.

Clearly, our thoughts, or the way we interpreted the weather, greatly affected the way we felt. A state of relaxed bliss turned into nervous anxiety even though the weather itself had not changed.

REMEMBER

People's total reaction to events consists of physiological responses, thoughts, and behaviors. Most feelings are adaptations to what is really happening. However, some problematic emotions stem from misinterpretations, misperceptions, and misguided reactions to events.

Distinguishing Thoughts from Feelings

Psychologists often query their clients to find out how they feel about recent events in their lives. Frequently, clients answer with how they *think* about the events rather than how they *feel.* Others know how they feel but are stumped when it comes to what they're thinking. In the next section, we discuss why people often end up out of touch with their feelings, thoughts, or both. Then, we discuss how to tune up your thoughts and feelings.

Blocking the blues

People often have trouble identifying and labeling their feelings and emotions, especially negative ones. Actually, the difficulty makes sense for two reasons.

First, emotions often hurt. No one wants to feel profound sadness, grief, anxiety, or fear. One simple solution is to *avoid* feelings entirely, and many creative ways to avoid emotion are available. Unfortunately, most of these methods can be destructive:

>> **Workaholism:** Some folks work all the time rather than think about what's disturbing them.

>> **Alcoholism and drug abuse:** When people feel bad, numbing their emotions with drugs and alcohol provides a temporary, artificial emotional lift; of course, habitually doing so can lead to addiction, ill health, and sometimes, even death.

>> **Denial and repression:** One strategy for not feeling is to fool yourself by pretending that nothing is wrong. Denial is often thought to be a conscious process, whereas repression is done outside of people's awareness, but the result is pretty much the same.

>> **Sensation seeking:** High-risk activities, such as sexual promiscuity and compulsive gambling, can all push away distress for a while.

>> **Distraction:** Athletics, entertainment, hobbies, television, scrolling through social media, and many other activities can cover up bad feelings. Unlike the preceding strategies, distraction can be a good thing. It's only when distractions are used in excess to cover up and avoid feelings that they become problematic.

The second reason that identifying, expressing, and labeling feelings is such a struggle for people is that they're taught from an early age that they "shouldn't" feel certain feelings. Parents, teachers, friends, and relatives bombard kids with "don't feel" messages. See the following examples of "don't feel" messages that you've probably heard before:

>> Big boys don't cry; don't be a baby!

>> You shouldn't feel that way!

>> Get over it!

>> It couldn't possibly hurt that bad.

>> Don't be a scared chicken.

>> Stop crying or I'll give you something to cry about!

That many people are described as "out of touch with their feelings" is no wonder. The problem with the habitual tendency to avoid feelings is that you don't find out how to cope with or resolve the underlying issue. Chronic avoidance creates a certain kind of low-level stress that builds over time.

Getting in touch with your feelings

Noticing your emotions can help you gain insight and discover how to cope more effectively. If you don't know what your feelings are, when they occur, and what brings them on, you can't do much about changing them.

To illustrate problems with identifying feelings, we turn to Dr. Patel and her patient, Jim, who is struggling with his marriage.

Dr. Patel: How did you feel when your wife said you were irresponsible?

Jim: I thought she was really out of line.

Dr. Patel: I see. But how did you *feel* about what she said?

Jim: She's at least as irresponsible as I am.

Dr. Patel: I suppose that's possible. But again, what were your *feelings,* your emotional reaction to what she said? Were you anxious, even angry, or upset?

Jim: Well, I couldn't believe she could accuse me of that.

Dr. Patel: I wonder if we should take some time to help you get in touch with your feelings?

Perhaps Jim is extremely anxious and worried that his wife will leave him, or he may be angry with her. Maybe her stinging criticism hurt him. Whatever the feeling, both Jim and Dr. Patel could find out plenty from knowing what emotion accompanies his upset.

This example shows that people may not always know how to describe what they're feeling. If you don't always know what you're feeling, that's okay. We realize that some people are aware of their feelings and know all too well when they're feeling the slightest amount of anxiety or worry. If you're one of those, feel free to skip or skim the rest of this section.

If you need to become more aware of your feelings, you can start immediately. Take some time right now to assess your mood. Then ask yourself what *feeling* captures the essence of those sensations. Of course, at this moment, you may not have any strong feelings. If so, your breathing is rhythmic, and your posture relaxed. Even if that's the case, notice what it feels like to be calm. At other times, notice your stronger sensations.

Feeling words describe your physical reaction to events and the labels you use to describe them.

REMEMBER

The following vocabulary list describes anxious feelings. The next time you can't find the right words to describe how you feel, one or more of these words may get you started:

Afraid	Obsessed
Agitated	Out of it
Anxious	Panicked
Apprehensive	Scared
Disturbed	Self-conscious
Dread	Shaky
Fearful	Tense
Frightened	Terrified
Insecure	Timid
Intimidated	Uneasy
Jittery	Uptight
Nervous	Worried

We're sure that we've missed a few dozen possibilities on the word list, and maybe you have a favorite way to describe your anxiety. That's fine. What we encourage you to do is to start paying attention to your feelings and bodily sensations. You may want to look over this list a number of times, and ask yourself whether you've felt any of these emotions recently. Try not to make judgments about your feelings. They may be trying to tell you something.

REMEMBER

Bad feelings only cause problems when you feel bad chronically and repeatedly in the absence of a clear threat. Anxiety and fear also have a positive function: They alert your mind and body to danger and prepare you to respond (see Chapter 3 for more on the fight-or-flight concept). For example, if the Joker knocks on your door, adrenaline floods your body and mobilizes you to either fight or run like your life depends on it, because it does! That's good for situations like that. But if you feel like the Joker is knocking on your door on a regular basis and he's not even in the neighborhood, your anxious feelings cause you more harm than good.

REMEMBER

Whether or not the Joker is knocking at your door, identifying anxious, fearful, or worried feelings can help you deal with them far more effectively than avoiding them. When you know what's going on, you can focus on what to do about your predicament more easily than you can when you're sitting in the dark.

Getting in touch with your thoughts

Just as some people don't have much of an idea about what they're feeling, others have trouble knowing what they're thinking when they're anxious, worried, or stressed. Because thoughts have a powerful influence on feelings, psychologists like to ask their clients what they were thinking when they started to feel upset. Sometimes, clients describe feelings rather than thoughts. For example, Dr. Baker had the following dialogue with Susan, a client who had severe anxiety:

> **Dr. Baker:** So, when your supervisor reprimanded you, you said you felt panicked. What thoughts went through your mind?
>
> **Susan:** Well, I just felt horrible. I couldn't stand it.
>
> **Dr. Baker:** I know; it must have felt really awful. But I'm curious about what thoughts went through your mind. What did you say to yourself about your supervisor's comments?
>
> **Susan:** I felt my heart pounding in my chest. I don't think I really had any thoughts actually.
>
> **Dr. Baker:** That's possible. Sometimes our thoughts escape us for a while. But I wonder, if you think about it now, what did those comments mean to you? What did you think would happen?
>
> **Susan:** I'm shaking right now just thinking about it.

As this example illustrates, people don't always know what's going on in their heads when they feel anxious. Sometimes you may not have clear, identifiable thoughts when you feel worried or stressed. That's perfectly normal.

The challenge is to find out what the stressful event *means* to you. That will tell you what your thoughts are. Consider the prior example. Susan may have felt panicked because she feared losing her job, or she may have thought the supervisor's criticism meant that she was incompetent. The boss's reprimand may have also triggered memories of her abusive father. Knowing what thoughts stand behind the feelings can help both Dr. Baker and Susan plan the next step.

Tapping your triggers

TIP

You may not always know what's going on in your mind when you feel anxious. To figure it out, you need to first identify the *situation* that preceded your upset. Zero in on what had just transpired moments before your troublesome feelings. Perhaps you

>> Opened your mail and found that your credit card balance had skyrocketed

>> Heard someone say something that bothered you

>> Worried that you might catch something awful because someone near you sneezed

>> Read the deficiency notice from your child's school

>> Wondered why your partner was so late coming home

>> Got on the scales and saw a number you didn't like

>> Noticed that your chest felt tight, and your heart was racing for no clear reason

On the other hand, sometimes the anxiety-triggering event hasn't even happened yet. You may be just sitting around and *wham* — an avalanche of anxiety crashes through. Other people wake up at 4 a.m. with worries marching through their minds. What's the trigger then? Well, it can be an image or a fear of all sorts of future events. See the following examples of anxiety-triggering thoughts and images:

>> I'll never have enough money for retirement.

>> Did I turn off the stove before I left the house?

>> We'll never finish writing this book on time!

>> No one is going to like my speech tomorrow.

>> I wonder if my new boss is a racist.

>> What if I get laid off next week?

>> What if my partner leaves me?

TIP

When you get upset or anxious, take a moment to reflect. Ask yourself what event just occurred or what thoughts or images floated into your mind just before you noticed the anxiety. Bingo! You'll see what triggered your anxious feelings. After you see how to capture your anxious thoughts in the next section, we show you how to put thoughts and feelings all together.

Snaring your anxious thoughts

If you know your feelings and the triggers for those feelings, you're ready to start looking at your thoughts in a new way. Thoughts powerfully influence emotions. An event may serve as the trigger, but it isn't what directly leads to your anxiety. It's the *meaning* that the event holds for you, and your thoughts reflect that meaning.

For example, suppose your spouse is 45 minutes late coming home from work. You may think *anxious* thoughts:

>> Maybe she's had an accident.

>> She's probably having an affair.

>> She must be at the bar again.

Or, you may have different thoughts that don't cause anxiety at all:

>> I love having time alone with the kids.

>> Oh, great I can surprise her by getting dinner on the table.

>> I like having time alone to work on house projects.

>> Traffic must be really bad tonight.

REMEMBER

Some thoughts create anxiety; others feel good; and still others don't stir up much feeling at all. Capturing your thoughts and seeing how they trigger anxiety and connect to your feelings is important. If you're not sure what thoughts are in your head when you're anxious, you can do something to find them.

TIP

First, focus on the anxiety trigger — the event or image that seemed to set things off. Think about it for a while; don't rush it. Then, ask yourself some questions about the trigger. The following list of what we call *minding-your-mind questions* can help you identify your thoughts or the meaning that the event holds for you:

>> Specifically, what about this event do I find upsetting?

>> What's the worst that could happen?

>> How might this event affect my life?

>> How might this affect the way that others see me?

>> Does this remind me of anything in my past that bothered me?

>> What would my parents say about this event?

>> How might this affect the way that I see myself?

Andrew's story illustrates how the questions about a triggering event can help clarify the nature of how one's thoughts influence feelings.

> **Andrew** loves his work. He manages computer systems and designs web pages for small businesses in his community. Andrew believes in hands-on service and often visits his clients just to see whether things are running smoothly. One Friday, Andrew pulls up to one of the law firm offices he's working for and sees three police cars parked by the front door. Andrew's heart races, and he perspires profusely at the mere sight of police. He feels terrified but doesn't know for sure what he's thinking.

In order to capture what's going on in his head, he answers a few of the minding-your-mind questions:

>> **Specifically, what about this event do I find upsetting?**

Something violent may be going on. I've always been afraid of violence.

>> **How might this event affect my life?**

I could get killed.

>> **How might this affect the way that others see me?**

Other people will think I'm a foolish coward.

>> **How might this affect the way I see myself?**

Like the coward I've always thought I was.

Andrew merely saw three police cars in front of a law office. Can you see where his mind took this event? Although workplace violence does occur, many other interpretations of this event are actually more likely. Nevertheless, Andrew needs to know what thoughts are running through his head when he feels anxious if he's going to be able to change how he responds to events like these.

TIP

When you work with the minding-your-mind questions, use your imagination. Brainstorm, and take your time. Even though Andrew's example doesn't answer all the questions, you may find it useful to do so.

Looking at the Feeling Cycle in Action

Once you understand what emotions consist of, it's time to figure out what causes you to feel those feelings. Monitoring your thoughts, feelings, and whatever triggers your anxiety paves the way for change. This simple strategy helps you focus on your personal pattern of stress and worry. The very act of paying attention brings your thinking process to light. This clarification helps you gain a new perspective.

Try using a Feeling Cycle Chart like the one in Table 5-1 to connect your thoughts, feelings, and anxiety triggers. When you monitor the triggers, include the day, time, place, people involved, and what was going on. When you record your anxious thoughts, use the minding-your-mind questions in the "Snaring your anxious thoughts" section earlier in this chapter. Finally, write down your anxious feelings and physical sensations.

TABLE 5-1   **Feeling Cycle Chart**

Anxiety Triggers	Anxious Thoughts	Feelings & Sensations
Tuesday morning on the way to work I heard a police siren in the distance.	I worried that a dangerous hot pursuit was in progress behind me.	Anxious, fearful, heart racing
At work on Wednesday I heard a sharp crashing sound.	I jumped and thought either a gun had gone off or something horribly destructive had occurred.	Jumpy and startled
I had to walk through a dark parking lot on Friday evening.	I imagined being mugged by someone jumping out from behind almost every car I passed by.	Tense, rapid breathing

To show you how to use the chart, we've filled it in with Andrew's notes that he took for a few days after starting therapy for his anxiety about violence.

TIP

You can use this simple technique to monitor your anxious feelings, thoughts, and triggers. Simply design your own Feeling Cycle Chart using the headings of Table 5-1. Keep track and look for patterns. Sometimes, just becoming more aware of your feelings, thoughts, and triggers softens your anxiety.

REMEMBER

If recording your thoughts, feelings, and triggers makes you more anxious, that's okay. It's common. Many other techniques in this book should help, especially the ones for challenging your thoughts in Chapter 6. But if the techniques in this book don't help you, consider seeking professional help.

Chapter **6**

Rethinking Your Thoughts

t's summer in New Mexico. There's a heat wave going on. The monsoon rains that usually cool us off in the evenings haven't yet started. We walk the dog every morning. During this heat wave, if we don't get out by 7 a.m., it gets pretty hot. This is Sunday morning; we dawdled over the paper, and it's almost 7:45. Here's what we're thinking:

> "We shouldn't have read the paper before walking. We could have read the paper after, and it wouldn't be so hot. If we don't walk for 30 minutes, our exercise routine is ruined. We'll be out of shape in no time. And fat, too. If we don't walk today, we'll probably start skipping our walks all of the time. Then, we'll be unhealthy, and maybe our cholesterol will go up as well as our blood pressure. And if we don't get our walk in, it will be hard to get going on writing today. We'll be in a bad mood again. How did we ever get so lazy?"

Meanwhile, our dog Ollie is waiting for his leash. We ask him if he wants to go for a walk. He jumps straight up and throws his body against the nearest leg. His answer seems to be yes. He's not worried about the heat or distressed about the time. He'll enjoy the walk. Language can ruin a perfectly good walk.

In this chapter, we review how thoughts (a form of internalized language) profoundly affect emotions and feelings in addition to behavior. Everyone can learn from dogs. Dogs don't ruminate or dwell on past regrets or future possible negative outcomes. Rather, dogs focus on the present moment.

Unlike dogs, humans think, interpret, and predict. However, you can train your mind to challenge unhelpful, inaccurate thoughts that contribute to anxiety and emotional distress. The following sections give you tools for rethinking thoughts.

Tackling Your Thoughts

When you feel anxious, take a moment and think about what you are thinking. Here's what we mean in a few examples:

>> **Andre** has a date. He's feeling very nervous. So, what is he thinking? He's thinking that his date (who he's never met) will think he's unappealing and socially inept.

>> **Juan** plans a cross-country road trip to visit an old friend. He has spent the last week obsessively worried about what could go wrong. He also worries about everyday events like entertaining friends, planning for retirement, or working on just about any project at home.

>> **Luna** had two panic attacks last year. She has the opportunity to go to a Broadway play she's wanted to see for a long time. She declines the invitation because her thoughts tell her she'll feel trapped in the theatre and may lose control, causing a humiliating commotion.

How do Luna, Juan, and Andre deal with their feelings and thoughts? We have three simple strategies for tackling anxious thoughts:

>> **Searching for evidence:** Looking at thoughts objectively and sifting through data and facts.

>> **Rethinking risk:** Recalculating the odds of anxious thoughts coming true — most people overestimate the odds.

>> **Imagining worst-case scenarios:** Reexamining the ability to cope — if, in fact, the worst does occur. Most folks underestimate their coping resources.

Tracking anxious thoughts and events is an important step in working on anxiety. But the following strategies take you further — by examining your thoughts and testing them out with logic and reason, you can relate to your thoughts in a different way. By challenging your thinking, you may find yourself less anxious.

TIP

The goal is not to stop thinking anxious thoughts, or for that matter, to stop having any anxious feelings. We want you to keep thinking and feeling. However, we want you to believe less in your thoughts and realize that feeling a bit anxious is not the end of the world. It's a different way of relating to thoughts and feelings that is the desired result.

Weighing the evidence

The thoughts that lead to your anxious feelings have most likely been around a long time. Most people consider their thoughts to be true. They don't question them. You may be surprised to discover that many of your thoughts don't hold up under scrutiny. If you carefully gather and weigh the evidence, you just may find that your thoughts rest on a foundation of sand.

TIP

Keep in mind that gathering evidence when you're feeling really anxious isn't always easy to do. At those times, it's hard to consider that your thoughts may be inaccurate. When that's the case, you're better off waiting until you calm down before hunting for the evidence. At other times, you may be able to find evidence right away if your anxiety isn't too out of control.

TIP

You can evaluate the validity of your thoughts by first jotting down an anxiety-arousing thought that you notice running through your mind. Write it down or dictate it into a device. Then, collect evidence that either supports the likelihood of your thought being true or disputes the likelihood of your anxious thought being true. Use the following questions to come up with disputing evidence:

>> Have I had thoughts like these at other times in my life? Have my dire predictions come true?

>> Do I have experiences that would contradict my thoughts in any way?

>> Is this situation really as awful as I'm making it out to be?

>> A year from now, how much concern will I have with this issue?

>> Am I thinking this will happen just because I'm feeling anxious and worried? Am I basing my conclusion mostly on my feelings or on the true evidence?

>> Am I assuming something without any solid evidence for my negative thought?

REMEMBER

Feelings are always valid in the sense that you feel what you feel, but they're not evidence for supporting anxious thoughts. For example, if you feel extremely anxious about taking a test, the anxiety is not evidence of how you will perform.

These evidence-gathering questions can help you discover evidence against your anxious or worrisome thoughts, because an anxious mind already knows the evidence that supports anxious thoughts.

To see how this works, you may recall that Andre (in the introduction to this section) was nervous about his upcoming date. Andre feared his date would find him unappealing and socially inept. First, Andre filled out the evidence supporting his anxious thought, which he found easy to do. Then, he used the evidence-gathering questions in this section to list the evidence against his anxious thoughts in the second column of the table.

After completing the task, Andre makes a new judgment about his anxious thought. He realizes that the evidence supporting his anxious thought doesn't hold up to scrutiny. He understands that his worry and stress about dating has a long history that isn't grounded in reality. He realizes that he has had many fun dates and just has to keep searching to find the right person. He still has anxious thoughts and still feels anxious before dates, but he worries less about his worries.

Consider filling out your own chart so that you can weigh the evidence carefully. Use the same column headings and format shown in Table 6-1. Be creative, and come up with as much evidence for and against your anxious thoughts as you can.

TABLE 6-1 ## Weighing the Evidence

Anxious Thought: I think my date will think I'm a loser and unappealing.	
Evidence Supporting My Anxious Thoughts	Evidence Against My Anxious Thoughts
One time I went on a date, and she said she had to go home unexpectedly. I never saw her again.	I have had at least a dozen dates with women who seemed interested, but I didn't really like them.
My ex-wife said I'd never find someone to love me.	Since my divorce, I have had two long-term relationships with attractive partners. One of them always called me sexy.
I think I am fairly unattractive.	I don't seem to have any trouble getting women to go out on a second date. If I were pathetic, that wouldn't happen.
I never know the right words to say.	Most of the time I don't really have too much trouble keeping a conversation going; I just worry about it too much.

Don't forget to use the evidence-gathering questions listed earlier in this section if you need help generating ideas.

Make a decision as to whether you truly think your anxious thoughts hold water. If they don't, you just may start taking them less seriously, and your anxiety could drop a notch or two.

Although charting your anxious thoughts and weighing the evidence just once may prove to be helpful, practice magnifies the effect. Mastering any new skill always requires practice. The longer you stay at it and the more times you chart your anxious thoughts versus the real evidence, the more benefit you'll gain.

Rethinking risk

Another important way to challenge your anxious thoughts is to look at how you assess the likelihood that an event may occur. When you feel anxious, like many people, you may *overestimate the odds* of unwanted events actually occurring. It's easy to do. For example, when was the last time you heard a news bulletin reporting that no one got bitten by a snake that day, or that millions of airplanes took off and landed and not a single one crashed? No wonder people overestimate disaster. Because disasters grab attention, people tend to focus on dramatic events rather than routine ones. That's why it's useful to think about the real, objective odds of your predicted catastrophe.

Thoughts are just thoughts. Subject them to a reality test.

When you find yourself making negative predictions about the future — such as the horrible time you'll have at a party, your odds of failing a test, or the likelihood that you'll end up in financial ruin — ask yourself the following reassessment of risk questions:

>> How many times have I predicted this outcome, and how many times has it actually happened to me?

>> How often does this happen to people I know?

>> If someone I know made this prediction, would I agree?

>> Am I assuming this will happen just because I fear that it will, or is there a reasonable chance that it will really happen?

>> Would people pay me to predict the future?

>> Do I have any experiences from my past that would suggest my dire prediction is unlikely to occur?

In addition to asking these questions, whenever possible, look up the statistical evidence as it relates to your fears. Of course, you can't always find statistics that help you. Nevertheless, the answers to the preceding questions will help you reassess your true risk and stop habitually making catastrophic predictions about the future.

Juan, who we wrote about in the beginning of this chapter, was always worried about things going wrong. The following story shows how Juan overestimates the probability of a horrible outcome.

> **Juan** rudely grabs the pan from his wife, Linda. He snaps at her, "I'll finish browning the meat. Go ahead and set the table." His abrupt demeanor stings Linda's feelings, but she knows how anxious he gets when company comes over for dinner. Juan tightly grips the pan over the stove, watching the color of the meat carefully. He feels irritable and anxious, "knowing" that the dinner will turn out badly. He frets that the meat is too tough and that the vegetables look soggy from overcooking. The stress is contagious, and by the time the company arrives, Linda shares his worries.

What outcome does Juan predict? Almost every time that he and Linda entertain, Juan believes that the food they prepare will be terrible, their guests will be horrified, and he'll be humiliated. The odds of this outcome can't be looked up in a table or a book. So how can Juan assess the odds realistically? Naturally, he answers the reassessment of risk questions and starts to change his anxious thoughts.

In doing so, Juan comes to realize that he and his wife have never actually ruined a dinner, although he has predicted it numerous times before. Furthermore, he tested his second prediction that his guests would feel horrified if the dinner did turn out badly. He recalled that one time he and Linda attended a barbeque where the meat was burned to the extent that it was inedible. Everyone expressed genuine sympathy and shared stories about their own cooking disasters. They ended up ordering pizza and considered it one of the more enjoyable evenings they'd spent in a long time. The hosts, far from humiliated, basked in the glow of goodwill.

Luna, also from the beginning of the chapter, worries about having a panic attack at a Broadway play. When she looks at the odds, she realizes that she's never had a panic attack at any theater performance, movie, or sports event. With this new information, she's ready to take the small risk and enjoy herself at the theater. She still has anxiety but believes it's worth moving ahead with her plans. Recalculating risk allows her to do that.

WHAT ARE THE ODDS?

We are all going to die (last time we checked). So, you have a 1 in 1 chance of eventually dying of something. Now, let's get more specific. Over a lifetime in the United States, the odds of being struck by lightning are about 1 in 180,000. The lifetime odds of being killed by a few other means in the United States are as follows:

- By a dog: About 1 in 119,000
- By a bee or a wasp: About 1 in 54,000
- Air travel: Too few deaths to make meaningful predictions!
- By a firearm: About 1 in 300
- Accidental gun discharge: About 1 in 9,100
- In an auto accident: About 1 in 110
- Choking on food: About 1 in 2,600
- Suicide: About 1 in 85
- Heart disease: About 1 in 6

Notice how the actual odds don't match very well with what people fear most. Many more people *fear* thunderstorms, snakes, spiders, and flying in airplanes than driving a car or being killed by a firearm. It doesn't make a lot of sense, does it? Finally, we should note that your individual odds may vary. If you regularly stand outside during thunderstorms, holding your golf clubs in the air, your chances of being struck by lightning are a little higher than average.

Deconstructing worrisome scenarios

Even faced with the evidence of the unlikelihood of the events you fear happening, you may be thinking that bad things still do, in fact, happen. Lightning strikes. Bosses hand out bad evaluations. Airplanes crash. Some days are just "bad hair days." Ships sink. People stumble and get laughed at. Some lose their jobs. Lovers break up.

The world gives us plenty of reasons to worry. Recalculating the true odds often helps. But you may still be stuck with the what-if worry — what if your concern truly happens? First, we show you how to cope with smaller, everyday worries, and then we address worst-case scenarios.

Small-potatoes scenarios

What do people worry about? Most of the time they worry about inconsequential, *small-potatoes scenarios.* In other words, outcomes that, while unpleasant, hardly qualify as life threatening. Nevertheless, these small scenarios manage to generate remarkable amounts of stress, apprehension, and worry.

Listen to what's worrying Gerald, Sammy, and Carol. Their stories illustrate common concerns that lead some people to feel highly anxious.

> **Gerald** worries about many things. Mostly, he worries about committing a social blunder. Before parties, he obsesses over what to wear. Will he look too dressed up or too casual? Will he know what to say? What if he says something stupid and people laugh? As you can imagine, Gerald feels miserable at social events. When he walks into a crowd, he feels as though a spotlight has turned his way, and everyone in the room is staring at him. He imagines that people not only focus on him but that they also judge him negatively.

> **Sammy** worries as much as Gerald; he just has a different set of worries. Sammy obsesses over the idea that he'll lose control and have to run away from wherever he is. If he's sitting in a classroom, he wonders whether he'll get so anxious that he'll have to leave, and of course, he assumes everyone will know why he left and think something is terribly wrong with him. If he's at a crowded shopping mall, he's afraid he'll "lose it" and start screaming and running out of control.

> **Carol** is a journalist. She feels anxiety almost every day. She feels pressure in her chest when each deadline approaches and dreads the day when she fails to get her story in on time. Making matters worse, she sometimes has writer's block and can't think of the next word to type for 15 or 20 minutes; all the while, the clock advances and the deadline nears. She's seen colleagues lose their jobs when they consistently failed to reach their deadlines, and she fears meeting the same fate one day. It's hard for Carol to stop thinking about her deadlines.

What do Gerald, Sammy, and Carol have in common? First, they all have considerable anxiety, stress, and tension. They worry almost every single day of their lives. They can't imagine the horror of dealing with the possibility of their fears coming true. But, more importantly, they worry about events that happen all the time and that people manage to cope with when they do.

Gerald, Sammy, and Carol all underestimate their own ability to cope. What if Gerald spills something at a party and people around him notice? Would Gerald fall to the floor unable to move? Would people point and laugh at him? Not likely. He'd probably blush, feel embarrassed, and clean up the mess. The party and Gerald's life would go on. Even if a few rude people laughed at Gerald, most would forget the incident and certainly wouldn't view Gerald any differently.

Sammy panics over the possibility that his feelings may overwhelm him. He worries that he'll have to run from wherever he is and look foolish in doing so. The fact that this has never happened to him doesn't stop Sammy's worrying.

Carol, on the other hand, has a bigger worry. Her worst-case scenario involves losing her job. That sounds serious. What would she do if she lost her job?

TIP

Whether you experience small- or medium-sized worries (small- or medium-potato scenarios), you can use the following *coping questions* to discover your true ability to cope. The answers to these questions help you deal with your own worst fears.

1. **Have I ever dealt with anything like this in the past?**
2. **How much will this affect my life a year from now?**
3. **Do I know people who've coped with something like this, and how did they do it?**
4. **Do I know anyone I could turn to for help or support?**
5. **Can I think of a creative new possibility that could result from this challenge?**

Carol, who worried about losing her job, turns to these questions to help her come to terms with her fears. Carol writes these answers to the coping questions:

1. **Have I ever dealt with anything like this in the past?**

   No, I've never lost a job before. This first question doesn't help me discover any better ways of coping, but it does help me see the possibility that I've been overestimating the risks of losing my job.

2. **How much will this affect my life a year from now?**

   If I did lose my job, I'd probably have some financial problems for a while, but I'm sure I could find another job.

3. **Do I know people who've coped with something like this, and how did they do it?**

   Well, my friend Janet lost her job a few months ago. Janet got unemployment checks and asked her parents for a little assistance. Now she has a new job that she really likes.

4. **Do I know anyone I could turn to for help or support?**

   I'd hate to do it, but my brother would always help me out if I really needed it.

5. **Can I think of a creative new possibility that could result from this challenge?**

When I think about it, I really sort of hate these daily deadlines at the newspaper. I do have a teaching certificate. What with the shortage of teachers right now, I could always teach high-school English and have summers off. Best of all, I could use those summers to write the novel I've always dreamed about writing. Maybe I'll quit my job now and do that!

It's amazing how often asking yourself these questions can eliminate the catastrophic consequences you associate with your imagined worry scenarios. Answering these questions can help you see that you can deal with the vast majority of your worries — at least the small- to medium-sized potatoes. But how about the worst-case scenarios (the really, really big potatoes)? Could you cope with real disasters?

Worst-case scenarios

Some peoples' fears involve issues that go way beyond social embarrassment or temporary financial loss. Severe illness, death, terror, natural disasters, disfigurement, major disabilities, and loss of a loved one are worst-case scenarios. How would you possibly cope with one of these? We're not going to tell you it would be easy, because it wouldn't be.

Marilyn's mother and grandmother both died of breast cancer. She knows her odds of getting breast cancer are higher than most. Almost every day of her adult life, she worries about her health. She insists on monthly checkups, and every stomach upset, bout of fatigue, or headache becomes an imagined tumor.

Her stress concerns both her family and her physician. First, her doctor helps her see that she is overestimating her risk. Unlike her mother and grandmother, Marilyn goes for yearly mammograms, and she performs regular self-exams. Not only that, she exercises regularly and eats a much healthier diet than her mother or grandmother did.

Marilyn realistically has a chance of getting breast cancer. How would she possibly cope with this worst-case scenario? You may be surprised to discover that the same questions used to deal with the small-potatoes scenarios can help you deal with the worst-case scenarios. Take a look at how Marilyn answered our five coping questions:

1. **Have I ever dealt with anything like this in the past?**

Unfortunately, yes. I helped my mother when she was going for chemotherapy. It was horrible, but I do remember laughing with her when her hair fell out. I understand chemotherapy isn't nearly as bad as it used to be. I never felt closer to my mother than during that time. We talked out many important issues.

2. **How much will this affect my life a year from now?**

Well, if I do get breast cancer, it will have a dramatic affect on my life a year from now. I may still be in treatment or recovering from surgery.

These first two questions focus Marilyn on the possibility of getting cancer. Even though she obsesses and worries about cancer, the intensity of the anxiety has prevented her from ever contemplating how she would deal with cancer if it actually occurred. Although she certainly hates the thought of chemotherapy or surgery, after she imagines the possibility, she realizes she could probably cope with them.

The more you avoid a fear, the more terrifying it becomes.

REMEMBER

3. **Do I know people who've coped with something like this, and how did they do it?**

Of course, my mother died of breast cancer. But during the last three years of her life, she enjoyed each moment. She got closer to all her kids and made many new friends. It's funny, but now that I think about it, I think she was happier during that time than any other time I can remember.

4. **Do I know anyone I could turn to for help or support?**

I know of a cancer support group in town. And my husband and sister would do anything for me.

5. **Can I think of a creative new possibility that could result from this challenge?**

I never thought of cancer as a challenge; it was a curse. But I guess I realize now that I can choose to be anxious and worried about it or just take care of myself and live life fully. If I do get cancer, I can hopefully help others like my mother did, and I'll use the time I have in a positive way. Besides, there's a good chance that I could beat cancer, and with medical advances, those chances improve all the time. I realize that I've spent so much time these past years worrying about getting cancer that I've neglected my family and life itself. I vow that I won't wait until my final days to get close to my family. It's time to start living right now, today.

TIP

When you have anxiety about something dreadful happening, it's important to stop avoiding the end of the story. Go there. The more you avoid contemplating the worst, the bigger the fear gets. In our work, we repeatedly found that our clients came up with coping strategies for the worst-case scenario, even the big stuff. Consider George's case.

George fears flying. He recalculates the risks of flying and realizes they're low. He says, "I know it's relatively safe and that helps a little, but it still scares me." Recently, George got a promotion. Unfortunately for George, the new position requires considerable travel. George's worst nightmare is that the plane will crash. George asks himself our coping questions and answers them as follows:

1. **Have I ever dealt with anything like this in the past?**

   No, I've obviously never been in a plane crash before.

2. **How much will this affect my life a year from now?**

   Not much, I'd be dead!

3. **Do I know people who've coped with something like this, and how did they do it?**

   None of my friends, relatives, or acquaintances has ever been in a plane crash.

4. **Do I know anyone I could turn to for help or support?**

   Obviously not. I mean, what could they do?

5. **Can I think of a creative new possibility that could result from this challenge?**

   How? In the few minutes I'd have on the way down, it's doubtful that many creative possibilities would occur to me.

Hmm. George didn't seem to get much out of our coping questions, did he? These questions don't do much good for a small number of worst-case scenarios. For those situations, we have the *ultimate coping questions*, followed by George's responses to these questions:

1. **What is it about this eventuality that makes you think you absolutely could not cope and could not possibly stand it?**

   Okay, I can imagine two different plane crashes. In one, the plane would explode, and I probably wouldn't even know what happened. In the other, something would happen to the engine, and I'd experience several minutes of absolute terror. That's what I really fear.

2. **Is it possible that you really could deal with it?**

> Could I deal with that? I guess I never thought of that before; it seemed too scary to contemplate. If I really put myself in the plane, I'd probably be gripping the seat, maybe even screaming, but I guess it wouldn't last for long. I suppose I could stand almost anything for a short while. At least if I went down in a plane, I know my family would be well taken care of. When I really think about it, as unpleasant as it seems, I guess I could deal with it. I'd have to.

Most people fear dying to some extent — even those with strong religious convictions (which can help) rarely welcome the thought. Nevertheless, death is a universal experience. Although most people would prefer a painless, quick exit during sleep, many deaths aren't as easy.

If a particular way of dying frightens you, actively contemplating it works better than trying to block it out of your mind. If you do this, you're likely to discover that, like George, you can deal with and accept almost any eventuality.

WARNING

If you find yourself getting exceptionally anxious or upset by such contemplation, professional help may be useful.

Cultivating Calm Thinking

Anxious thoughts capture your attention. They hold your reasonable mind hostage. They demand all your calmness and serenity as ransom. Thus, when you have anxious thoughts, it helps to pursue and destroy them by weighing the evidence, reassessing the odds, and reviewing your true ability to cope (see the previous sections for the how-tos).

Another option is to crowd out your anxious thoughts with calm thoughts. You can accomplish this task by using one of three techniques. You can try what we call the friend perspective; you can construct new, calm thoughts to replace your old, anxious thoughts; or you can try positive affirmations.

Considering a "friend's" perspective

Sometimes, simple strategies work wonders. This can be one of them. When your anxious thoughts hold most of your reasonable mind hostage, you still have a friend in reserve who can help you find a fresh perspective. Where? Within yourself.

TIP

Try this technique when you're all alone — alone, that is, except for your friend within. Truly imagine that a good friend is sitting across from you and talk out loud. Imagine that your friend has exactly the same problem that you do. Take your time, and really try to help your friend. Brainstorm with your friend. You don't have to come up with instant or perfect solutions. Seek out every idea you can, even if it sounds foolish at first — it just may lead you to a creative solution. This approach works because it helps you pull back from the overwhelming emotions that block good, reasonable thinking. Don't dismiss this strategy just because of its simplicity!

Julian's example demonstrates this technique in action.

> **Julian** worries about his bills. He has a charge card balance of a few thousand dollars. His car insurance comes due in a couple of weeks, and he doesn't have the money to pay for it. When Julian contemplates his worry, he thinks that maybe he'll go broke, his car will be repossessed, and eventually, he'll lose his house. He feels he has no options and that his situation is hopeless. Julian loses sleep because of his worry. Anxiety shuts down his ability to reason and analyze his dilemma.
>
> Now, we ask Julian to help an old friend. We tell him to imagine Richard, a friend of his, is sitting in a chair across from him. His friend is in a financial bind and needs advice on what to do. Richard fears he will lose everything if he can't come up with some money to pay his car insurance. We ask Julian to come up with some ideas for Richard.
>
> Surprising to Julian, but not to us, he comes up with a cornucopia of good ideas. He tells Richard, "Talk to your insurance agent about making payments monthly rather than every six months. Also, you can get an advance on your credit card. Furthermore, isn't there an opportunity to do some overtime work? Talk to a credit counselor. Couldn't one of your relatives loan you a few hundred dollars? In the long run, you need to chip away at that credit-card debt and pull back a little on your spending."

Creating calm

Another way to create calm thoughts is to look at your anxious thoughts and develop a more reasonable perspective. The key with this approach is to put it on paper. Leaving it in your head doesn't do nearly as much good.

This strategy doesn't equate with mere positive thinking, because it doesn't help you create a Pollyanna alternative — that is, a thought that is unrealistically optimistic. Be sure that your reasonable perspective is something that you can at least partially believe in. In other words, your emotional side may not fully buy into your alternative view at first, but the new view should be something that a reasonable person would find believable.

TIP

Your task will be easier if you've already subjected your anxious thinking to weighing the evidence, rethinking the risk, and reevaluating your coping resources for dealing with your imagined worst-case scenarios, as we describe in earlier sections.

Table 6-2 provides some examples of anxious thoughts and their reasonable alternatives. We also provide you with a Pollyanna perspective that we *don't* think is useful.

TABLE 6-2   Developing a Reasonable Perspective

Anxious Thought	Reasonable Alternative	Pollyanna Perspective
If I wear a tie and no one else does, I'll look like an idiot.	If no one else wears a tie, some people will no doubt notice. However, they probably won't make a big deal out of it. Even if a couple of people do, it really won't matter to me at all a few weeks from now.	Everyone will think I look great no matter what!
If I get a C on this exam, I'll be humiliated. I have to be at the top of my class. I couldn't stand it if I weren't.	If I get a C, I certainly won't be happy. But I'll still have a good grade average and a good chance at a scholarship. I'll just work harder the next time. I'd love to be at the top of my class, but life will go on just fine if I fall short of that.	There's no way that I won't get an A. I must, and I shall.
If I lose my job, in a matter of weeks I'll be bankrupt.	If I lose my job, it will cause some hardship. However, odds are good I'll find another one. And my wife has offered to increase her hours to help out if I need her to.	I could never lose my job!
I'd rather walk up 20 flights of stairs than take this elevator. The thought of the doors closing terrifies me.	It's time I tackled this fear, because the odds of an elevator crash are infinitesimally small. Taking the elevator is pretty scary, but perhaps I can start by just riding up or down a couple of floors and work my way on from there.	I need to quit being such a wimp. I'm just going to jump on this thing and take it to the top!

WARNING

We showed you the Pollyanna perspective because it's important not to go there. You may think the last example of the Pollyanna perspective — getting over your fear in an instant — looks great. That would be nice, we suppose, if only it worked that way. The problem with that approach is that you set yourself up for failure if you try it. Imagine someone truly terrified of elevators trying to jump on and take it to the top floor all at once. More likely than not, the person would do it that one time, feel horror, and make the fear even worse.

Be gentle with yourself; go slowly when confronting your anxious thoughts and fears.

REMEMBER

Watching Out for Worry Words

Think about the mental chatter that goes on in your mind. Do you ever exaggerate? Put yourself down? Predict horrible outcomes? For example, if your computer is acting up, do you get angry at yourself, predict that you'll never get anything done, and surmise that the day will surely be ruined? Those inner conversations can stir up a whirlwind of anxiety. The next sections help you discover what words contribute to your anxiety. They come in several forms and categories, and we show you how to track these words down. Then we offer strategies for finding alternative words and phrases to quell your unnecessary anxiety.

Stacking sticks into bonfires of anxiety

"Sticks and stones can break my bones, but words can never hurt me." Perhaps you heard this saying as a child. Parents often try to assuage their kids' hurt feelings through this catchphrase, but it usually doesn't work because words do have power. Words can frighten, judge, and hurt.

If those words came only from other people, that would hurt enough. But the words that you use to describe yourself, your world, your actions, and your future may have an even greater impact on you than what you hear from others. The example of Jason and his wife Beverly illustrates this point. What starts out as a simple conversation between husband and wife leads to lots of anxiety and marital stress.

> **Jason's wife Beverly,** who's a little worried about her husband's blood pressure, mentions at breakfast that it looks like he's gained a little weight. "Oh, really?" Jason queries.
>
> "Maybe just a little bit; it's no big deal. I just worry about your health," she replies.
>
> Over the course of the next few hours, Jason starts ruminating about what his wife said. "I'm a *pig* . . . She's *totally disgusted* with me . . . She'll *never* want to have sex with me again . . . Losing weight is *impossible* for me . . . I'm *certain* that she'll leave me; that would be *unbearable.*"

By the afternoon, Jason feels intense anxiety and tension. He's so upset that he withdraws and sulks through the rest of the day. Beverly knows something's wrong and worries that Jason is losing interest in her.

What happened? First, Beverly delivered a fairly mild statement to Jason. Then, rather than ask Beverly for clarification, Jason pounded himself with a slurry of anxiety-arousing words — *pig, totally disgusted, never, impossible, certain,* and *unbearable.* Jason's mind overflowed with powerful words that grossly distorted Beverly's original intention. His inner thoughts no longer had any connection to reality.

WARNING

The worry words that you use inflame anxiety easily and are rarely supported by evidence or reality. They become bad habits that people use unwittingly. However, we have good news: Like any habit, the anxiety-arousing word habit can be broken.

Worry words come in four major categories. In the upcoming sections, we go through each of them with you carefully:

» **Extremist:** Words that exaggerate or turn a minor event into a catastrophe

» **All-or-none:** Polar opposites with nothing in between

» **Judging, commanding, and labeling:** Stern evaluations and name-calling

» **Victim:** Underestimating your ability to cope

Encountering extremist words

It's amazing how selecting certain words to describe events can literally make mountains out of molehills. Extremist words grossly magnify or exaggerate troubling situations. In doing so, they aggravate negative emotions. Read about Emily, who turns a fender bender into a catastrophe.

Emily, pulling out of a tight parking spot at the grocery store, hears metal scraping metal. Her bumper dents a side panel of a late-model SUV parked next to her. Emily stomps on the brake, jams her car into park, and leaps out to inspect the damage — a 4-inch gash.

Using her cellphone, she calls her husband, Ron. Hysterical, she cries, "There's been a *horrible* accident. I *destroyed* the other car. I feel *awful;* I just *can't stand it.*" Ron attempts to calm his wife and rushes to the scene from work. When he arrives, he's not that surprised to find the damage to be quite minor. He's well aware of Emily's habit of using extreme words, but that doesn't mean Emily isn't upset. She is. Neither she nor Ron realizes how Emily's language lights the fuse for her emotional response.

Most of Emily's problematic language falls under the category of extremist words. The following list gives you a small sample of extremist words: *agonizing, appalling, awful, devastating, disastrous, horrible,* and *unbearable.*

Of course, reality can be horrible, appalling, and downright awful. It would be hard to describe the Holocaust, September 11th, famine, or our worldwide pandemic in milder terms. However, all too often, extremist words like these reshape reality. Think about how many times you or the people you know use these words to describe events that, while certainly unpleasant, can hardly be described as earth-shattering.

REMEMBER

Life presents challenges. Loss, frustration, aggravation, and pain routinely drop in like annoying, unwelcome guests. You may try to banish them from your life, but your best efforts won't keep them from stopping by — uninvited as usual. When they arrive, you have two choices. One is to magnify them, and tell yourself how *horrible, awful, unbearable,* and *intolerable* they are. But when you do that, you only manage to intensify your anxiety and distress. Your other option is to think in more realistic terms. (See the "Exorcising your extremist words" section, later in this chapter, for more on realistic options.)

Misrepresenting with all-or-none, black-or-white words

Pick up any black-and-white photograph. Look carefully, and you'll see many shades of gray that likely dominate the picture. Most photos contain very little pure black or white at all. Calling a photo black-and-white oversimplifies and fails to capture the complexity and richness of the image. Just as calling a photograph black-and-white leaves out many of the details, describing an event in black-and-white terms ignores the full range of human experience. Like a photograph, little of life is black or white.

Nevertheless, people easily slip into language that oversimplifies. Like extremist language, this all-or-nothing approach intensifies negative feelings. The following example shows how categorizing life in all-or-nothing terms can lead to upset feelings.

> **Thomas** puts his newspaper down, unable to concentrate, and tells his wife that he'd better get going. "I didn't sleep a wink last night. I've been *totally* freaked about my sales quota this month. I'll *never* make it. There's *absolutely* no way. Sales *entirely* dried up with the slower economy, but the boss has *zero* tolerance for extenuating circumstances. I'm *certain* he's going to jump my case. It would be *absolutely* impossible to find another job if he fires me."

Thomas distorts reality by declaring that he'll *never* make the sales quota. Then his anxiety escalates. In the process, he concentrates on the negative rather than searching for positive solutions. If Thomas is at a loss for additional all-or-none words, he can borrow from the following list: *all, always, ceaseless, complete, constant, everyone, forever, invariably, no one, none* . . . you get the idea.

REMEMBER

Few things (other than death, taxes, and change) occur with absolute certainty. You may recall pleading with your parents for a later curfew. We bet you told them that *everyone* stays out later than you. If so, you did it for good reason, hoping that the word *everyone* would make a more powerful statement. Nevertheless, your parents probably saw right through your ploy. Everyone oversimplifies sometimes; our language has many words for distorting reality. (For an all-or-none antidote, see the "Disputing all-or-none" section later in this chapter.)

Running into judging words

You *must* read this book more carefully than you have been. Not only that, but you *should* have read more of it by now. And you *should* have taken the exercises more seriously. You're a *pathetic jerk. Shame* on you!

We're just kidding.

What authors in the world would take their readers to task like that? None that we can think of. That sort of criticism is abusive. People react with dismay when they witness parents humiliating their children by calling them *stupid* or *rotten*. Many would view a teacher who calls his students *fools* and describes their best effort as *awful* or *pathetic* as equally abusive. That kind of harsh judgment hardly inspires; berating crushes the will.

However, many people talk to themselves this way or even worse. Some hear a steady stream of critical commentary running through their minds. You may be your own worst critic. Many folks take the critical voice that they heard in childhood and turn it on themselves, often magnifying the critique in the process. Critical words come in three varieties, although they overlap, and sometimes a particular word can belong in more than one category:

>> **Judgments:** These are harsh judgments about yourself or what you do. For example, when you make a human mistake and call it an utter failure, you're judging your actions rather than merely describing them. Words like *bad, inadequate, stupid, pathetic,* or *despicable* are judgments.

>> **Commandments:** This category contains words that dictate absolute, unyielding rules about your behavior or feelings. If you tell yourself that you *should* or *must* take a particular action, you're listening to an internal drill

sergeant. This punishing drill sergeant tolerates no deviation from a strict set of rules.

>> **Labels:** Finally, self-critical labels put the icing on the cake. Words like *loser, pig, monster, jerk,* and *failure* come to mind as disturbing labels people sometimes put on themselves like a name tag worn at a party.

See the later section "Judging the judge" for ways to replace these words with more positive language.

Turning to victim words

You may remember the story *The Little Engine That Could* by Watty Piper, about the train that needed to climb a steep hill. The author of the book wisely chose not to have the engine say, "I think I *can't;* I'll never be able to do it; this hill is impossible."

The world feels like a much scarier place when you habitually think of yourself as a victim of circumstance. Certain words can serve as a flag for that kind of thinking, such as these victimizing words: *can't, defenseless, frail, helpless, impossible, impotent, incapacitated, overwhelmed, powerless,* and *vulnerable.*

WARNING

Victim words demoralize. They offer no hope. Without hope, there's little reason for positive action. When victims believe themselves defenseless, they feel vulnerable and afraid.

However, people who describe themselves as victims do enjoy a few advantages: They don't feel compelled to do much about whatever predicaments they face; people express sympathy for them; and some people offer to take care of them. Yet these advantages become self-defeating in the long run. To help yourself overcome the victim mind-set, flip to the later section "Vanquishing victim words."

Refuting and Replacing Your Worry Words

Ask yourself how you truly want to feel. Few people like feeling anxious, worried, and stressed. Who would choose those feelings? So, perhaps you agree that you prefer to feel calm and serene rather than wound up.

A good way to start feeling better is to change your worry words. However, you aren't likely to stop using worry words just because we told you that they create anxiety. That's because you still may think that these words accurately describe you and/or your world. Many people go through life without questioning their self-talk, simply assuming words equate with reality.

TIP

In order to refute the accuracy of your internal chatter, consider a small change in philosophy. This shift in philosophy entails questioning the idea that thoughts, language, and words automatically capture truth. Then substitute that idea with a new one, using logic and evidence-gathering to structure your reality. At the same time, keep in mind that your goal is to take your internal dialogues less seriously.

In the following sections, we look at each category of worry words and show you how to replace them with words that more accurately represent the situation.

Exorcising your extremist words

The vast majority of the time when people use extremist words, such as *intolerable, agonizing, horrible, awful, hopeless,* and *ghastly,* they use them to describe everyday events. When you hear yourself using those words, subject them to a logical analysis.

For example, few events in life are unbearable. After all, you've managed to get through every single difficult time in your life up to now or you wouldn't be alive and reading this book. Many circumstances feel really bad, but somehow, you deal with them. Life goes on.

TIP

When you think in extreme terms, such as *unbearable, intolerable, can't stand it, awful,* and *disastrous,* you lose hope. Your belief in your ability to manage and carry on diminishes. Consider whether your unpleasant experiences are actually described more accurately in a different way:

>> Difficult but not unbearable

>> Uncomfortable but not intolerable

>> Disagreeable but not devastating

>> Distressing but not agonizing

When you drop extreme language from your vocabulary, your emotions also often drop. Moderate descriptors soften your reactions. Less-extreme portrayals lead you to believe in your ability to cope. Humans have a surprising reservoir of resilience. You cultivate your capacity for problem-solving and survival when you have hope.

Disputing all-or-none

People use all-or-none words, such as *never, always, absolute, forever, unceasing,* and *constant,* because they're quick and easy, and they add emotional punch. But these terms have insidious downsides: They push your thinking to extremes, and your emotions join the ride. Furthermore, all-or-none words detract from coping and problem-solving.

TIP

Rarely does careful gathering of evidence support the use of all-or-none words. Many people use all-or-none words to predict the future or to describe the past. For example, "I'll *never* get promoted," or, "You *always* criticize me." Whether you're talking to yourself or someone else, these words hardly produce calmness, nor do they describe what has happened or what's likely to happen in the future. So try to stay in the present. Table 6-3 illustrates the switch between all-or-none words and calm, evidence-gathering words that keep you *in the present without distortion.*

TABLE 6-3   ## Switching to the Present

All or None	In the Present without Distortion
I'll never get promoted.	At this moment, I don't know whether I'll be promoted. However, I'll do everything that I can to see to it that it happens.
You always criticize me.	Right now, your criticism makes me feel bad.
I always panic when I'm in a crowd.	Right now, I can't know for certain whether I'll panic the next time I'm in a crowd. I may panic, and I may not. If I do, it's not the worst thing in the world, and I won't die from it.

Judging the judge

Words that judge, command, or label, such as *should, must, failure, fool, undeserving,* and *freak,* inflict unnecessary pain and shame on their recipients. You may hear these words from others or from your own critic within.

Labels and judgments describe a person as a whole, but people usually use them to describe a specific action. For example, if you make a mistake, you may say to yourself, "I can't believe that I could be such an *idiot!*" If you do, you just made a global evaluation of your entire being based on a single action. Is that useful? Clearly, it's not accurate, and most importantly, the judgment doesn't lead you to feel calm or serene.

Like the other types of worry words, commandments don't inspire motivation and improved performance. Yet people use these words for that very purpose. They think that saying "I *must* or *should*" will help them, but these words are more likely to make them feel guilty or anxious. Self-scolding merely increases guilt and anxiety, and guilt and anxiety inevitably decrease both motivation and performance.

TIP

Try replacing your judging, commanding, and labeling words with more reasonable, accurate, and supportable alternatives. Consider the following examples:

>> **Judging:** I got a pathetic score on my LSAT test. I must be too stupid to become a lawyer.

Reasonable alternative: It wasn't the score that I wanted, but I can study more and retake it.

>> **Commanding:** I must have a happy marriage. I should have what it takes to keep it happy.

Reasonable alternative: Much as I'd like to have a happy marriage, I was okay before I met my wife, and I can learn to be okay again if I have to. Being happily married is just my strong preference, and I don't have complete control over the outcome — it does take two, after all.

Vanquishing victim words

Victim words, such as *powerless, helpless, vulnerable, overwhelmed,* and *defenseless,* put you in a deep hole and fill you with a sense of vulnerability and fear. They make you feel as though finding a way out is impossible and that hope remains out of reach. Yet as with other worry words, only rarely do they convey absolute truth.

Nevertheless, victim words can become what are known as self-fulfilling prophecies. If you *think* a goal is impossible, you're not likely to achieve it. If you *think* that you're powerless, you won't draw on your coping resources. As an alternative, consider the logic of your victim words. Is there anything at all that you can do to remedy or at least improve your problem?

TIP

Gather evidence for refuting victim words that appear in your self-talk. Ask yourself whether you've ever managed to cope with a similar situation before. Think about a friend, an acquaintance, or anyone at all who has successfully dealt with a burden like yours.

After you consider the logic and the evidence, ask whether victim words make you feel better, calmer, or less anxious. If not, replace those words with new ones, as in the following examples:

>> **Victim:** I have a fatal disease, and I'm totally powerless to do anything about it.

Reasonable alternative: I have a disease that's indeed often fatal. However, I can explore every avenue from new experimental treatments to alternative treatments. If that doesn't work, I can still find meaning with the rest of my life.

>> **Victim:** I feel overwhelmed by debt. I feel helpless and have no options other than declaring bankruptcy.

Reasonable alternative: I do have considerable debt. However, I could go to a credit-counseling agency that specializes in renegotiating interest rates and payments. I may also be able to get a second, part-time job and chip away at the bills. If I ultimately do have to declare bankruptcy, I can slowly rebuild my credit.

Chapter **7**

Busting Up Your Anxious Assumptions

Some people love to speak in front of crowds; others shake at the very thought of public speaking. Ever notice how people respond to criticism? Some blow it off, some get angry, and others are extremely embarrassed. While one person may become anxious about traffic, airplanes, or health, another becomes anxious about finances, and still another feels anxious only around bugs. A few people rarely become anxious at all.

This chapter explains why different people respond to the same event in extremely different ways. We show you how certain beliefs or assumptions about yourself and the world cause you to feel the way you do about what happens. One way to think about these beliefs is to think of them as lenses or glasses that you look through. As you know, sometimes lenses can be cloudy, dirty, smoky, cracked, or distorted, making the world look dark, gloomy, and dangerous. Other lenses are rose-colored or clear, reflecting either an optimistic or realistic perspective.

Dark or distorted lenses make people scared or anxious when they look at the world through them. Those who consistently look through distorted lenses develop biased viewpoints of reality. We label those warped viewpoints anxious assumptions. We show you how certain anxious assumptions generate excessive worry and anxiety. These beliefs come primarily from your life experiences — they don't mean you're defective. Of course, as discussed in Chapter 3 and elsewhere, all aspects of anxiety are also influenced by biological factors. The questionnaire in this chapter helps you discover which assumptions may agitate and create anxiety in you. We provide ways for you to challenge those anxious assumptions. Replacing your troubling assumptions with more reasonable appraisals can reduce your anxiety.

Understanding Anxious Assumptions

An assumption is something that you presume to be correct without question. You don't think about such assumptions or core beliefs; rather, you take them for granted as basic truths. For example, you probably believe that fall follows summer and that someone who smiles at you is friendly and someone who scowls at you isn't. You assume without thinking that a red light means stop and a green light means go. Your assumptions provide a map for getting you through life quickly and efficiently.

And that's not necessarily a bad thing. Your assumptions guide you through your days with less effort. For example, most people assume their paychecks will arrive more or less on time. That assumption allows them to plan ahead, pay bills, and avoid unnecessary worry. If people didn't make this assumption, they'd constantly check with their payroll department or boss to ensure timely delivery of their checks to the annoyance of all concerned. Unfortunately, the core belief of expecting a paycheck is shattered when jobs are scarce or layoffs increase. Understandably, people with expectations of regular paychecks feel pretty anxious when their assumptions don't hold true.

Similarly, most people have assumptions about food. They assume that the food sold in the grocery store is safe to eat — in spite of occasional news reports about tainted food showing up in stores. On the other hand, food sold on a street corner in a third-world country might be assumed to be less safe to eat. Many tourists would avoid such food even if the food was actually fine. So, while people act on their assumptions, they're not always correct in doing so.

As you can see, sometimes assumptions fail to provide useful information. They may even distort reality so much that they arouse considerable distress. For example, before giving a speech, you may tremble, quiver, and sweat. You may worry that you'll stumble over your words, drop your notes, or even worse, faint from fear. Even though these things have seldom happened when you've previously given speeches, you always assume that they will this time. That dread of embarrassment comes from an anxious assumption that when you have to perform, you will likely mess up and be embarrassed.

REMEMBER

Anxious assumptions assume the worst about yourself or the world — and usually they're incorrect.

When activated, anxious assumptions cause anxiety and worry. Unfortunately, most people don't even know they have them. Therefore, anxious assumptions can go unchallenged for many years, leaving them free to fuel anxiety.

Sizing Up Anxious Assumptions

Perhaps you're curious as to whether you hold any anxious beliefs or assumptions. People usually don't even know that they have these troubling beliefs, so they don't question them. Challenging these assumptions has to start with knowing which ones you have. In the following sections, we identify five anxious assumptions and then provide a quiz to help you determine whether you suffer from any of them.

Recognizing anxious assumptions

Five major anxious assumptions capture much of what people worry about:

>> **Perfectionism:** Perfectionists assume that they must do everything right or they will have failed totally, and the consequences will be devastating. They ruminate over minor details.

>> **Approval:** Approval addicts assume they must win the approval of others at any cost to themselves. They can't stand criticism.

>> **Vulnerability:** Those afflicted with the vulnerability assumption feel at the mercy of life's forces. They worry all the time about possible disasters.

>> **Control:** Those with the control assumption feel that they can't trust or rely on anyone but themselves. They always want to be the driver — never the passenger.

>> **Dependency:** Those with the dependency assumption feel they can't survive on their own and turn to others for help.

These anxious assumptions powerfully influence the way you respond to circumstances. For example, imagine that the majority of comments you get on a performance review at work are quite positive, but one sentence describes a minor problem. Each assumption causes a different reaction:

>> **If you have the perfectionism belief,** you severely scold yourself for your failure. You won't even see the positive comments.

>> **If you have the approval assumption,** you obsess about whether your boss still likes you.

>> **If you have the vulnerability assumption,** you believe that you're about to lose your job, and then your house and car.

>> **If you have a control assumption,** you focus on how working for someone else makes you feel out of control and helpless.

>> **If you have the dependency belief,** you look to others for support and help. You ask your coworkers to intervene on your behalf with the boss.

Various individuals react completely differently to the same event, depending on which assumption those individuals hold. Just imagine the reaction of someone who simultaneously holds several of these core beliefs. One sentence in a performance review could set off a huge emotional storm of anxiety and distress.

You may have one or more of these anxiety-creating assumptions to one degree or another. Taking the quiz in the following section helps you find out which, if any, anxious beliefs you hold — whether you know it or not.

Assessing your anxious assumptions

In Table 7-1, place a check mark in the column marked "T" if a statement is true or mostly true as a description of you; conversely, place a check mark in the column marked "F" if a statement is false or mostly false as it pertains to you. Please don't mark your statement as "T" or "F" simply based on how you think you *should* be; instead, answer on the basis of how you really do act and respond to events in your life.

Most people endorse one or more of these items as true. So don't worry too much if you find quite a few statements that apply to you. For example, who doesn't hate being embarrassed? And most people worry at least a little about the future.

TABLE 7-1   # The Anxious Assumption Quiz

T	F	Perfectionism
		If I'm not good at something, I'd rather not do it.
		When I make a mistake, I feel terrible.
		I think if something's worth doing, it's worth doing perfectly.
		I can't stand to be criticized.
		I don't want to turn my work in to anyone until it's perfect.
T	*F*	*Approval*
		I often worry about what other people think.
		I sacrifice my needs to please others.
		I hate speaking in front of a group of people.
		I need to be nice all the time or people won't like me.
		I can rarely say no to people.
T	*F*	*Vulnerability*
		I worry about things going wrong.
		I worry a great deal about my safety, health, and finances.
		Many times, I feel like a victim of circumstances.
		I worry a great deal about the future.
		I feel pretty helpless much of the time.
T	*F*	*Control*
		I hate taking orders from anyone.
		I like to keep my fingers in everything.
		I hate to leave my fate in the hands of others.
		Nothing would be worse than losing control.
		I do much better as a leader than a follower.
T	*F*	*Dependency*
		I'm nothing unless someone loves me.
		I could never be happy on my own.
		I ask advice about most things that I do.
		I need a great deal of reassurance.
		I rarely do things without other people.

So, how do you know whether you have a problem with one of these assumptions? You start by looking at each assumption one at a time. If you checked one or more items as true, that raises the possibility that this assumption causes you some trouble. Just how much trouble depends on how much distress you feel.

Ask yourself what makes you feel especially anxious. Does it have to do with one or more items that you checked as true? If so, you probably struggle with that anxious assumption. We cover each anxious assumption and ways to overcome it later in this chapter.

WARNING

If you have a number of these assumptions, don't get down on yourself! You likely developed your anxious beliefs for good reasons. You should congratulate yourself for starting to figure out the problem. That's the first step toward feeling better.

WARNING

In some cases, core beliefs reflect real experiences from early in life, and those events continue to occur. For example, anxiety associated with racism likely formed because of learning throughout childhood and young adulthood. The anxiety has some protective benefit for dealing with the current racist world. Thus, changing a vulnerability assumption could be dangerous. That's because holding on to a certain amount of vulnerability may help a person of color stay prepared in the face of the unfortunate occurrence of racist incidents.

Coming Down with a Case of Anxious Assumptions

If you have too much anxiety, one or more anxiety-arousing core beliefs undoubtedly contribute to your problems. But it's especially important to know that you're not crazy for having anxiety-provoking assumptions! People acquire these beliefs in three completely understandable ways:

>> When experiences in childhood prevent the development of a reasonable sense of safety, security, acceptance, or approval

>> When chronic stressful events, while not traumatic, add up over time

>> When shocking, traumatic events shatter previously held assumptions

The following sections explain in more detail how these experiences lead to anxious assumptions.

Acquiring assumptions in childhood

You may have been one of the lucky ones who glided through childhood feeling loved, accepted, safe, and secure. Perhaps you lived in a home with two loving parents, a dog, a station wagon, and a white picket fence. Or maybe not. You probably didn't have a perfect childhood. Not many people do.

For the most part, your parents probably did the best they could, but they were human. Perhaps they had bad tempers or ran into financial difficulties. Or possibly, they had addictions or failed to look out for your safety as well as they should have. For these and numerous other reasons, you may have acquired one or more anxious assumptions.

The following example illustrates the most common time in life for anxious core beliefs to develop — childhood.

> **Tanner** developed his problematic assumption as a child. Tanner's mother rarely gave him much approval. She harshly criticized almost everything he did. For example, his room was never quite clean enough, and his grades were never quite stellar enough. Even when he brought his mother a gift, she told him it was the wrong color or size. He felt he could do almost nothing right.
>
> Slowly but surely, Tanner acquired an assumption — "I must be absolutely perfect, or I will be a total failure." Being perfect is pretty hard. So you can imagine why he now feels anxious most of the time.

Notice that Tanner's anxious belief about perfection didn't come about from a massive, single event. Rather, a series of criticisms and corrections built his need for perfection up over time. Unfortunately, his conviction that everything must be perfect continues to plague him as an adult.

REMEMBER

If you have anxious assumptions, you don't question them. You believe in them wholeheartedly. Just as Tanner assumes the sky is blue, he believes that he's either perfect or a complete failure. When Tanner undertakes a project, he feels intense anxiety due to his morbid fear of making a mistake. Tanner's anxious assumption is that of painful perfectionism, and it makes him miserable, but he doesn't know why.

Shattering your reasonable assumptions

Anxious assumptions most often begin during childhood (see the preceding section), but not always. Sometimes, what seems to be a common, though unfortunate, occurrence can lead to a new anxiety-arousing core belief. The following example illustrates how present-day life can create an anxiety-arousing assumption.

> **Bill** had always assumed, like most people do, that working hard and saving his money would assure him a safe, secure financial future and retirement. He has worked at his family's auto parts and service store for 25 years. He follows his financial advisor's advice and, at the age of 50, has half of his money in the stock market. The economy takes a horrible hit, and his shop lays off most of its employees. Bill reluctantly puts a substantial part of his savings into buoying the business. Then the stock market tanks, and Bill sees that his hard-won gains have virtually evaporated. Eventually, the store closes its doors, and Bill looks for work.
>
> At the age of 50, he sees that he's not likely to find something that pays what he used to get from the family business. Instead of looking at ways to develop new skills or options, he sits hopelessly watching the stock market on television for many hours every day.
>
> Bill, formerly confident and self-assured, feels insecure, worried, and obsessed about his financial status. He has formed a new assumption — a vulnerability belief focused on money. He worries constantly about how he'll get by financially.

Bill had a very good reason to form that assumption, and like most anxious assumptions, Bill's anxious belief contains some truth — you can never know with certainty what the future will bring. However, as with all anxious assumptions, the problem lies in the fact that Bill underestimates his ability to adapt and cope. Therefore, he now spends his days engaged in unproductive obsessing rather than changing his goals and lifestyle while developing new skills or possibilities.

Challenging Those Nasty Assumptions: Running a Cost/Benefit Analysis

After taking our quiz and finding out about anxiety-arousing beliefs in the previous sections, you now have a better idea about which ones may be giving you trouble. In the old days, many therapists would have told you that insight is enough. We disagree. Pretend you just took an eye test and found out that you suffer from severe nearsightedness. Wow, you have insight! But what does that change? Not much. You still walk around bumping into the furniture.

You're about to get a prescription for seeing through your problematic assumptions. It starts with a cost/benefit analysis. This analysis paves the way for making changes.

Perhaps you think your perfectionism assumption is good and appropriate. Maybe you believe that you have profited from your perfectionism and that it has helped you accomplish more in your life. If so, why in the world would you want to challenge or change it? The answer is simple. You wouldn't.

Therefore, you need to take a cold, hard look at the costs as well as any possible benefits of perfectionism. Only if the costs outweigh the benefits does it make sense to do something about your perfectionism. After looking at the examples in the next five sections, see the "Challenging your anxious assumptions" section for directions on how to conduct a cost/benefit analysis for your personal problematic anxious core beliefs.

Analyzing perfection

Knowing which problematic anxious assumptions lurk in your mind is the first step toward change. However, just knowing isn't going to get you there. You need to feel motivated to make changes. Change takes effort, and frankly, it's downright hard to change. The story about Prudence shows you how someone who believes she must be perfect finds the motivation to change her assumption through a cost/benefit analysis.

> **Prudence**, a successful trial attorney, works about 70 hours per week. Her closet is full of power suits; she wears her perfectionism like a badge of honor. Prudence works out to maintain her trim figure and manages to attend all the right social events. Too busy for a family of her own, she dotes on her 9-year-old niece and gives her lavish presents on holidays.
>
> Prudence is shocked when her doctor tells her that her blood pressure has gone out of control. Her doctor wonders about the stress in her life. She says it's nothing that she can't handle. He inquires about her sleep habits, and she replies, "What sleep?"
>
> Prudence is in trouble, and she doesn't even know it. She believes that her high income is due to her relentless standards and that she can't let up in the slightest way.
>
> Prudence has little hope of changing her firm conviction that she must be perfect if she doesn't face it head-on. Her doctor suggests that she see a counselor, who tells her to run a cost/benefit analysis of her perfection assumption.

A cost/benefit analysis starts with listing every imaginable benefit of any given assumption. Including every benefit your imagination can possibly conjure up is important. Then, and only then, should you start thinking about the costs of the assumption.

Prudence's fondness for her perfectionism is no small wonder. Filling out the benefits in her cost/benefit analysis is easy for her, but what about the costs? Review Table 7-2 for what she writes after she works at the task and consults friends and colleagues for ideas.

TABLE 7-2   Cost/Benefit Analysis of Prudence's Perfectionism

Benefits	Costs
My income is higher because of my perfectionism.	I don't have much time for fun.
I rarely make mistakes.	I'm anxious, and maybe that's why my blood pressure is so high.
I'm widely respected for my work.	I don't have many friends.
I always dress professionally and look good.	I spend too much time and money on clothes and makeup.
Other people admire me.	I get very irritable when people don't measure up.
I'm a role model for my niece.	Some people hate me for my harsh standards and expectations of them. I've lost several secretaries in the last six months.
	I hardly ever see my niece because I'm so busy.

REMEMBER

The cost/benefit analysis helps you to know whether you really want to challenge your assumptions. You would probably agree that Prudence's example shows more costs than benefits. But wait, it isn't finished. The final step is to examine carefully whether you would lose all the benefits by changing the assumption.

For example, Prudence attributes her high income to her dedication and long work hours. Perhaps she's partly right, but would her income evaporate if she worked just a little less? Most likely, if she worked less, her income might drop a bit, but with less anxiety, she might increase her efficiency enough to make up the difference. If she were less irritable, she would be able to retain her secretarial staff and gain efficiency there, too.

Would Prudence actually start making more mistakes if she relaxed her standards? Research suggests that excessive anxiety decreases performance. With respect to her niece, Prudence isn't really getting the benefit that she thinks she is, because she's not around enough to serve as an effective role model. Finally, more people fear Prudence than admire her. So you see, many times the perceived benefits of an assumption evaporate upon close inspection.

Tabulating approval

Approval addicts constantly crave admiration and acceptance from others. They worry about rejection and criticism. They constantly scan people's faces for any sign of disapproval. People with this anxious assumption often misinterpret the intentions of others. However, they're reluctant to give up their powerful belief in the need for approval. That's because they fear that letting go of their worry habit will result in abandonment or rejection.

> **Anne**, a graduate student in social work, has to meet each week with her advisor for supervision of her casework. She dreads those supervision sessions, always fearing her advisor's criticism. Anne does plenty for her clients; she does anything that she thinks they may need help with — spending hours of her own time, even running errands for them if they ask. Her supervisor tries to tell her to pull back from giving excessive help to her clients; he says that her bending over backwards to assist clients doesn't help her or her clients. She cries after hearing her supervisor's comments.
>
> However, Anne's worst fears surround the required presentations in front of graduate school classmates. Before giving talks to her classmates, she spends an abundance of time in the bathroom feeling ill. During lively discussions in her class, Anne remains quiet and almost never takes sides. Anne is addicted to approval.
>
> Anne walks quietly through life. People rarely criticize her. She avoids embarrassment by not taking risks. She is kind-hearted and people like her. What's wrong with that?

Well, a cost/benefit analysis of Anne's desperate need for approval reveals that people walk all over her. It also shows that fellow students fail to appreciate how bright she is, because she rarely speaks up in class. Anne neglects her own needs and at times feels resentful when she does so much for others, and they do so little to return the favor. Anne's approval addiction doesn't give her what she expects. Sure, she rarely receives criticism, but because she takes so few risks, she never gets the approval and praise that she really wants.

Reviewing vulnerability

People who unabashedly believe that they're constantly vulnerable worry about their safety, livelihood, and security. They traverse through their worlds in a state of constant, high alert. The following example illustrates someone with the vulnerability concern.

> **Peter,** a college graduate with a business degree, receives a promotion that requires him to move to California, but he turns it down because he fears big cities and earthquakes. Peter watches the weather channel and listens to the news

before he ventures any distance from home and avoids driving if the radio reports any chance of inclement weather. Peter's worry restricts his life. He also worries about his health and often visits his doctor, complaining of vague symptoms, such as nausea, headaches, and fatigue. Peter's doctor suggests that his worry may be causing many of his physical problems. He tells Peter to fill out a cost/benefit analysis of his belief that he is constantly at risk.

After completing his cost/benefit analysis on the issue of vulnerability, Peter realizes that he's spending a lot of time worried about things he has no control over. Although he avoids risk when possible, he realizes he's not living a full, happy life. Someone as entrenched as Peter in his vulnerability assumption certainly isn't going to give it up just because of his cost/benefit analysis. However, the analysis starts the ball rolling by showing him that his assumption is costing him big-time. The exercise motivates him to start thinking about doing some things differently.

Counting up control

People who have an anxious need for control only feel comfortable when they hold the reins. They fear that others won't do what's necessary to keep the world steady and safe. Giving up control makes them feel helpless. At the same time, many of those with this assumption fear losing control and embarrassing themselves if that were to happen.

> **Jeff,** the head of a division at his engineering company, likes order in his life. His employees know him as a taskmaster who micro-manages. Jeff takes pride in the fact that, although he asks for plenty, he demands more of himself than he does of his employees. He issues orders and expects immediate results. His division leads the company in productivity.
>
> You may think that Jeff has it made. It certainly sounds like his issue with control pays off handsomely. But scratch beneath the surface, and you see a different picture. Although known for productivity, his division is viewed as lacking in creativity and leads all others in requests for transfers. The real cost of Jeff's control assumption comes crashing down upon him when, at 46 years of age, he suffers his first heart attack.

Jeff has spent many years feeling stressed and anxious, but he has never looked closely at the issue. Jeff's quest for control nets him the opposite of what he wanted. Ultimately, he loses control of his life and health.

If control is one of your problematic assumptions, do a cost/benefit analysis. Jeff's fate doesn't have to be yours, too.

Debating dependency

People who believe they're dependent on others turn to friends and family whenever the going gets even a little tough. They don't see themselves as capable. They believe they need others to help them get through almost any difficulty. Unfortunately, people with such neediness often lose the people they depend on the most. Why? They burn them out. The next story about Daniel is typical.

> **Daniel** lived with his parents until, at 31 years of age, he married Dorothy. He met Dorothy online and, after just a few dates, decided to marry her. Dorothy seemed independent and secure, qualities that Daniel craved but lacked. At the beginning of their relationship, Dorothy was fond of Daniel's constant attention. Today, he still calls her at work three or four times every day, asking for advice about trivia and sometimes seeking reassurance that she still loves him. If she's five minutes late, he's beside himself. He often worries that she'll leave him. Dorothy's friends tell her that they aren't sure that Daniel could go to the bathroom by himself. Daniel believes that he can't survive without her. After he quits several jobs because "they're too hard," Dorothy threatens divorce. Daniel finally sees a therapist who has him conduct a cost/benefit analysis of his dependency issues, as shown in Table 7-3.

TABLE 7-3   ## Cost/Benefit Analysis of Daniel's Dependency

Benefits	Costs
I get people to help me when I need it.	I never find out how to handle difficult problems, tasks, situations, and people.
Other people take care of me.	Sometimes people resent having to take care of me.
Life isn't as scary when I have someone to lean on.	My wife hates me calling her all the time.
It's not my fault when problems arise or plans don't work out.	My wife gets angry when I don't take initiative.
I'm never lonely because I always make sure that I have someone around.	I might drive my wife away if I continue to cling to her so much.
It makes life easier when someone else takes care of business.	Sometimes I'd like to take care of something, but I think I'll screw it up.
	I haven't discovered how to master very much. Sometimes I feel like a mama's boy.

Someone like Daniel is unlikely to give up his defective dependency assumption without more work than this. However, a cost/benefit analysis can provide an initial push. Meaningful change takes time and work.

Challenging your anxious assumptions

You can run your own cost/benefit analysis. See the list of assumptions in the "Sizing Up Anxious Assumptions" section, earlier in this chapter. Which ones trouble you? Do you tend toward perfection, seeking approval, vulnerability, control, or dependency or maybe have a combination of these core beliefs? Take your time. Ponder and accumulate as many perceived benefits and costs as you can for each belief. When you're finished, ask yourself if you feel just a bit more ready to do something about these problematic assumptions.

REMEMBER

Anxiety-arousing assumptions often get you the *opposite* of what you want. They cause worry and stress, and rarely give you any true benefits. If you're going to give up your assumptions, you need to replace them with a more balanced perspective.

Designing Calm, Balanced Assumptions

So, do you think you have to be perfect or that everyone has to like you all the time? Do you always need to be in charge? Do you feel that you can't manage life on your own? Or, do you sometimes feel that the world is a dangerous place? These are the difficult assumptions that stir up worry, stress, and anxiety.

Another problem with these beliefs is that they do contain a kernel of truth. For example, it *is* nice when people like you, and it *is* nice to be in charge sometimes. We all need to depend on others sometimes as well. That sliver of truth makes people reluctant to abandon their assumptions.

The solution is to find new, balanced beliefs that hold even greater truth, but old assumptions are like habits — they're hard to break. To do so requires finding a new habit to replace the old one. It also takes plenty of practice and self-control, but it isn't that difficult. You just need a little persistence.

In the following sections, we go over each of the assumptions and help you see how to develop an alternative, more reasonable assumption to replace your old one. Try using these reasonable, balanced perspectives to talk back to your anxious assumptions when they occur. Finally, once you develop a new assumption, try acting in ways that are consistent with that new belief.

WARNING

If you find that your anxious assumptions rule your life and cause you intense anxiety and misery, you may want to consult a professional psychologist or mental health counselor. But first, start with your primary care doctor to rule out physical causes. Sometimes anxiety does have a physical base, and your primary care doctor can give you a referral after physical causes have been looked into. Should you consult a professional, you'll still find this book useful because most anxiety experts are familiar with the tools that we provide, and they'll help you implement them.

Tempering perfectionist tendencies

Perfectionists believe they have to be the best in everything they do. They feel horrible when they make mistakes, and if they're not outstanding at something, they generally refrain from trying. Fortunately, a good cost/benefit analysis can often help them see that perfectionism exacts a terrible toll.

But if not perfect, then what? Some people think it would mean going to the other extreme. Thus, if they weren't perfect, these folks assume that they would become sloths with no standards at all.

TIP

If you're worried about giving up on your perfectionism, we have good news for you. The alternative is not the other extreme! You may find it helpful to copy the following statements, or what we call "balanced views" on an index card. Or, you may want to think of your own alternatives. Just be sure they aim for the middle ground. Carry your card around with you as a reminder for those times when you start to get hung up on perfectionism.

>> I like to do well at things, but it's silly to think that I have to be the best at everything.

>> I'll never be good at everything, and sometimes it's really fun just to try something new.

>> Everyone makes mistakes; I need to deal with it when I do.

In other words, if you currently hold the assumption that you must be perfect and do everything right or you'll fail totally, try to think in less extreme terms. A more balanced viewpoint is that you like doing things well, but that *all humans make mistakes and so do you.* You don't want to be above the rest of us humans.

TIP

Collect evidence that refutes your perfectionism. For example, think about all the people you admire, yet who make numerous mistakes over time. When they make mistakes, do you suddenly see them as defective? Doubtful. Use the same standard for yourself.

THE DEADLY SECRETS OF PERFECTIONISM

Perfectionism pays off . . . sometimes. A little bit of perfectionism probably can improve the quality of your work, sports, and other endeavors as long as you don't let it get out of hand. How bad is it when perfectionism gets too extreme? Worse than you may think. Perfectionists often become extreme procrastinators just to avoid making mistakes. Not only that, perfectionists more often develop various types of anxiety disorders, depression, physical ailments, and eating disorders. Worst of all, it appears that adolescents who suffer from perfectionism have a higher rate of suicide.

Balancing an approval addict

Approval addicts desperately want to be liked all the time. They sacrifice their own needs in order to please others. Standing up for themselves is hard because to do so would risk offending someone. When criticized, even unfairly, they tend to fall apart.

But isn't it good to want people's approval? As with all anxious beliefs, it's a matter of degree. Taken too far, the approval assumption can ruin your life.

But if you quit worrying about getting people's approval, what will happen then? Will you end up isolated, rejected, and alone? Is rudeness and arrogant behavior the alternative to being nice all the time?

TIP

If you worry about giving up your approval addiction, we have an alternative. You just may want to carry these ideas in your pocket. Feel free to make up some on your own as well.

>> What other people think matters, but it's not usually crucial.

>> Some people won't like me no matter what I do. That's true for everyone.

>> I need to start paying attention to my needs at least as much as other people's.

TIP

In addition, consider collecting evidence that refutes your anxious need for approval. For example, think about people whom you like and admire who manage to speak their minds and look out for their own needs. Why do you like them? It's probably not because they bow and scrape to your every whim. Besides, someone who did that would probably turn you off.

If you feel addicted to approval and assume you must have the approval of others at all times and at virtually any cost, consider a more balanced perspective. Sure, everyone likes to be liked, but realize that no matter what you do, some people won't like you some of the time. Try thinking that your needs matter and that what other people think of you does not define your worth.

Balancing vulnerability

People who fervently believe in their vulnerability feel unsafe and worry constantly about every conceivable mishap. They may worry about safety, health, natural disasters, or the future; they often feel like victims of life's circumstances. They feel helpless to do much about their lot. The modern world with constant news about pandemics, natural catastrophes, financial ruin, and terror probably increases everyone's sense of vulnerability. It's no wonder that anxiety rates have skyrocketed.

People with this assumption fail to understand that worry has never stopped a single catastrophe. Nor does excessive worry help you prepare for the inevitable bad luck and misfortune that occur in everyone's life.

TIP

A better, alternative assumption can keep you reasonably safe without all that worry. If you want to give up your vulnerable assumption, try carrying these ideas with you and use them like mantras, repeating them to yourself frequently:

>> I need to take reasonable precautions but stop obsessing over safety. The amount of preparedness that I or anyone else can take action on is limited.

>> I will go to the doctor for an annual physical, pay attention to nutrition and exercise, and follow my doctor's advice. Beyond that, worrying about my health is pointless.

>> Some unfortunate mishaps are unforeseen and out of my control. I need to accept that bad things happen; worry is no shield.

TIP

Again, if you hold the vulnerability assumption and feel that you're at the mercy of life's dangerous forces, you may want to consider a more balanced point of view. Try thinking that no one can prevent the trials and tribulations of life, but that you can usually cope when they do occur. Collect evidence about the many unpleasant incidents that you were able to cope with in the past. For example, when you had high blood pressure, perhaps you exercised or took medication to control it, or when you lost someone whom you cared for, you grieved, but you survived.

Relaxing control

Some people always want to take charge. They can't stand taking orders. When in a group, they dominate the conversation. They always want to know everything that's going on around them in their families and at work. They don't delegate well. Some fear flying because they aren't in the cockpit.

Being a control freak is tiring and causes plenty of anxiety, too. Perhaps you have trouble with this anxious belief. Many highly successful, intelligent folks do, and this assumption isn't easy to give up. But the costs to health, well-being, and relationships are staggering.

TIP

As for all anxiety-arousing assumptions, we have an alternative, balanced view that will serve you better than control ever did. Review our suggestions. And if you must take control and rewrite them, that's okay, too!

> » I can usually trust other people to do what they need to do. I don't have to manage everyone, and they're likely to resent me if I do.

> » Asking for help or delegating a task isn't the end of the world, and sometimes, delegating is much more efficient.

> » I don't have to know every single detail of what's going on in order to feel in charge. Letting go reduces stress.

> » Letting others lead can make them feel better and take a load off me.

TIP

Think of a time in your life when someone else was in charge and things turned out pretty well anyway. In other words, collect evidence about when not having control has worked out.

Diminishing dependency

People who feel excessively dependent believe they can't make it on their own. They ask for advice when they don't really need it and seek reassurance that they're loved or that what they've done is right. The thought of not having a close relationship terrifies them. They can barely imagine trying to live life alone. You're not likely to find someone with a dependency assumption eating alone at a restaurant.

Many anxious assumptions ironically backfire. Excessively dependent people eventually annoy and irritate those whom they depend on. Partners of dependent people often distance themselves from the relationship after they become weary of constant clinging and helplessness.

TIP

If you battle with dependency, consider some of our alternative thoughts. Write these on an index card and keep them handy for frequent review. Feel free to embellish them or come up with some of your own.

>> It's nice to have someone who loves me, but I can survive on my own and have done so in the past.

>> Seeking advice can be useful; working through an issue on my own is satisfying.

>> I prefer to be with other people, but I can find out how to appreciate time alone.

If you buy into the defective dependency assumption — that you can't be all right on your own and that you need help with all that you do — try thinking in a more reasonable fashion. Realize that it's nice to have someone to depend on, but that you're capable of many independent actions.

TIP

Collect evidence of your capabilities. Do you put gas in your own car? Do you manage your own checkbook? Do you get to work and back on your own? Can you remember the times that you did well without someone? Realizing that you have taken independent action successfully and remembering that you have pulled yourself through many difficult spots all on your own can boost your confidence enough to help you take more independent action in the future.

Above All: Be Kind to Yourself!

Anxious core beliefs or assumptions are surprisingly common, and many successful people who don't even have a full-blown anxiety disorder tend to fall under the influence of one or more of these assumptions. Therefore, it's important that you don't beat up on yourself for "being under the influence."

The origins of your anxious assumptions could be in your childhood or the result of a traumatic event. Possibly your parents peppered you with criticism and that caused you to crave approval. Perhaps you had an unfortunate accident or trauma that caused you to feel vulnerable. Maybe your parents failed to provide you with consistent care and love, leading you to feel insecure, and, as a result, you yearn for help and affection. These represent merely a few of an infinite number of explanations for why you develop anxious assumptions. The point is that you did not ask for your problematic beliefs; you came by them honestly.

You've started on the road to overcoming anxiety. Go slowly; take pleasure in the journey and realize that change takes time and practice. Be patient with yourself.

Chapter **8**

Mindful Acceptance

Has your car ever been stuck on a muddy road? What happens if you gun the accelerator harder when the wheels start to spin? They spin even harder, the mud flies everywhere, and the rut gets deeper. Anxiety can be like that: The harder you try to break free, the more stuck you get.

In this chapter, we explain how to use *acceptance* as one way to get out of your anxiety trap. Threads of what we call *mindful* acceptance show up throughout this book. We weave the threads together to form a tapestry. We show how acceptance helps you stop spinning your wheels so you can calmly consider productive alternatives. We discuss how too much concern with ego and self-esteem can make seeing the way out difficult, and we explain how living in the present provides a roadway to a more balanced life. Finally, we give you some thoughts about the possible role of spirituality in finding serenity.

TIP

When you find yourself stuck in the rut of anxiety, don't slam down on the accelerator. Sit back, let the wheels settle a bit, rock back into the rut, and then gently push forward. Eventually, you'll discover a rhythm of going forward, then rocking back, and your efforts will lead you to solid ground.

Accepting Anxiety? Hey, That's a Switch!

So, why is it that after showing you how to get rid of your anxiety, we tell you to mindfully accept it? Have *we* lost our minds? Isn't this book supposed to be about *overcoming* anxiety?

Well, yes, of course we want you to overcome your anxiety. But the paradox of anxiety is that the more you feel you must rid yourself of it, the more anxious you feel. The more your anxiety disturbs you, the more it ensnares you.

Imagine going to a carnival or birthday party where someone gives you a Chinese handcuff — a little, decorative, woven straw tube. You put both index fingers into the tube. Then, you try to extract your fingers. The tube closes tightly around your fingers. The harder you pull, the tighter the handcuffs squeeze; a way out doesn't seem to exist. So, you pull even harder. Eventually, you realize that the only way out is to quit trying.

Anxiety mimics the squeezing of Chinese handcuffs. The more you struggle, the more trapped you feel. Insisting that your anxiety go away this second is a surefire way to increase it! Instead, sit back and think about your anxiety. We describe how in the following sections.

Taking a calm, dispassionate view

Anthropologists study the behavior and culture of human beings. They make their observations objectively from a dispassionate, scientific perspective. We want you to view your anxiety like an anthropologist — coolly detached.

TIP

Wait for the next time that you feel anxious. Study your anxiety and prepare a report that conveys what anxiety feels like in your body, how it affects your thoughts, and what it does to your actions. Don't judge the anxiety — just observe it. Then, being as objective as possible, answer the following questions in your report:

>> Where in my body do I feel tension? In my shoulders, back, jaw, hands, or neck? Study it and describe how the tension feels.

>> Are my hands sweating?

>> Is my heart racing? If so, how fast?

>> Do I feel tightness in my chest or throat?

>> Do I feel dizzy? Study the dizziness and describe it.

>> What am I thinking? Am I . . .

- Making negative predictions about the future?

- Making a mountain out of a molehill?

- Turning an unpleasant event into a catastrophe?

- Upset about something that's outside of my control?

>> What is my anxiety telling me to do?

- To avoid doing something that I want to do?

- That I need to be perfect?

- That I have to cover up my anxiety?

Mel's story that follows provides a good example of how your powers of observation may help you get a handle on your anxious feelings.

Mel, a 38-year-old hospital administrator, experienced his first panic attack three years ago. Since then, his attacks have increased in frequency and intensity, and he's even started to miss work on days when he feared having to lead staff meetings.

Now, he works with a therapist to decrease his panic. The therapist notices that Mel's perfectionism drives him to demand instant improvement. He reads everything he's assigned and tries to do every task perfectly. The therapist, realizing that Mel needs to slow down and back up, gives him an assignment to pretend that he's an anthropologist on a mission and to write a report about his anxiety. Mel completes the assignment as follows:

I started noticing a little shortness of breath. I thought: It's starting again! Then my heart began to race. I noticed it was beating fast and I wondered how long it would last. Then I noticed that my hands were sweating. I felt nauseous. I didn't want to go to work. I could almost hear the anxiety telling me that I would feel much better if I stayed home because if I went to work, I'd have to talk to a room full of upset surgeons. I have to tell them about the new billing procedures. They're not going to like it. They'll probably rip me to shreds. What an interesting image. I've never really been ripped into shreds, but my image is amazing! If I get too anxious, my words will turn into nonsense, and I'll look like a total fool. This is interesting, too. I'm making incredibly negative predictions about the future. It's funny — as I say that, I feel just a tiny bit less anxious.

Mel discovered that letting go and merely observing his anxiety helped. Rather than attack his anxious feelings and thoughts, he watched and pondered his experience by really trying to emulate the sense of scientific curiosity of anthropologists.

TIP

Simply observing anxiety like an anthropologist won't rid you of anxiety. That's not the point. However, doing so will help you to take a step back and start relating to your anxiety in a new way. Rather than seeing anxiety as horrible, terrible, and unacceptable, you can look at it more dispassionately.

Tolerating uncertainty

Anxious people usually detest uncertainty. If only they could control everything around them, they might not worry so much, and that's probably true: If you could control everything, you wouldn't have much cause for worry, would you?

The rather obvious flaw in this approach lies in the fact that life consists of constant uncertainty and a degree of chaos. In fact, a basic law of physics states that, even in so-called hard sciences, absolute certainty is nonexistent. Accidents and unforeseen events happen.

For example, you don't know the day and time that your car will break down on the way to work. You can't predict the stock market, although many people try. Bad things happen to good people all the time. Even if you spent every moment of your waking life trying to prevent illness, financial difficulties, and loss of loved ones, you couldn't do it.

Not only is the task of preventing calamities impossible, but you can easily ruin most of your present moments if you try. Think about it. If you check your car's engine before leaving for work each day, if you scrimp and save every possible penny for retirement, if you never eat ice cream because of the fat content, if you overprotect your children because you worry that they'll get into trouble, if you wash your hands every time you touch a doorknob (well, go ahead and wash during a pandemic), if you never take a risk, then what will your life be like? Probably not much fun.

REMEMBER

Worry doesn't change what will happen. Some people think that if they worry enough, bad things won't occur. Because bad things don't happen to them on most of those worry days, they feel like their worrying has paid off. But worry by itself has never in the history of humans prevented anything from happening. Not once.

Find out how to embrace uncertainty, which can make life both interesting and exciting. Discover how to appreciate adversity as well as a little suffering. Without some suffering and adversity, you fail to value the good moments.

When you find yourself feeling anxious, ask yourself whether your worry is an attempt to control the unpredictable. For example, many people worry about their retirement funds in the stock market. They watch how their stocks are doing every single day. They scan the newspaper for financial information that may possibly help them know when to sell at just the right moment. Yet, as the past few years have shown, there are no guarantees in the stock market.

Parents of teenagers are worry experts. They sit anxiously waiting for their sons and daughters to come in from nights out. They worry about drugs, alcohol, accidents, or other dangers. All of the worrying doesn't protect the kids. What does help are the efforts parents make throughout their kids' development, teaching them how to make good, safe decisions. Nighttime worry doesn't help keep kids safe, but it does make parents miserable. Have a cup of sleepy-time tea, and go to bed.

REMEMBER

Let go of your need to predict and control. Of course, take reasonable precautions regarding your health, family, finances, and well-being, but when worry about the future invades the present enjoyment of your life, it has gone too far. Appreciate uncertainty and live well today.

Being patient with yourself

When you think about patience, what comes to mind? Calm, acceptance, and tolerance. When you become anxious, try to be patient and kind with yourself and say to yourself,

>> Okay, I'm feeling anxious. That's my experience.

>> Like other feelings, anxiety comes and goes.

>> Let me be present with my anxiety.

In the example of Jeanine that follows, Jeanine's contrasting reactions, first with impatience and then with patience, provide an illustration of how you, too, can turn your impatience into patience.

Jeanine begins to feel anxious during the morning commute. She leaves home at 7:15 a.m. and usually can count on being to work on time at 8 a.m. Frequently, she arrives about five minutes early, but once a month or so, traffic backs up, and she's a few minutes late. This morning appears to be one of those.

The impatient Jeanine: Traffic is at a standstill, and anxiety churns in Jeanine's stomach and builds. Sweating and clutching the steering wheel, she begins tracking the ways that she can change lanes and get through a bit faster. She hates starting her day out like this. She can't stand the anxiety and tries to get rid of it, but she fails. She visualizes her boss noticing her tardiness and the others at her office looking up at her. Anxiety turns to anger as she criticizes herself for not leaving earlier.

The patient Jeanine: Traffic is at a standstill, and anxiety churns in Jeanine's stomach. Clutching the steering wheel, she fights the urge to change lanes. She notices and accepts the anxiety in her body, thinking, "I may be late, but most every morning, I am on time or early. My boss and co-workers know that. I can feel my anxiety, but that's my experience. How interesting. I'll arrive a few minutes late this morning, and that's okay."

In the second scenario, the anxiety dissipates because Jeanine allows herself to feel the present moment without judgment or intolerance. She connects to her present situation with patience.

REMEMBER

Like everything else, making patience a habit takes practice. You build your tolerance for patience over time. Like building muscles by lifting weights, you can build the patience muscles in your mind a little at a time.

Appreciating your imperfections

All too often, anxious people feel that they must be perfect in order for others to like and accept them. No wonder they feel anxious. Nobody's perfect, and no one ever will be. Take the case of Kelly.

Kelly is perhaps as close to perfect as you can find. Kelly always wears exactly the right fashionable clothes, the right colors, and her accessories always match. She takes classes in interior design, so her house has just the right look. She exercises four times a week and eats only healthy foods. Her makeup, which she applies with great care, appears flawless. She always knows just what to say, never stumbling over a single word or swearing. She always exhibits kindness and has a positive outlook.

Would you like to have a beer with Kelly? Does she seem like someone you'd like to hang out at a pool with on a summer weekend? Would you feel easy and natural around Kelly? Frankly, we'd probably pass on the idea of having her as one of our best friends.

Think about one of your good friends with whom you like to spend time, someone you enjoy and value, and someone you've known for a while. Picture that person in your mind, and recall some of the good times that you've spent together. Let yourself enjoy those images. Think about how much you appreciate this person and how your life has been enriched by the relationship.

Realize that you've always known about your friend's negative qualities and imperfections, yet you've continued to appreciate your friend. Perhaps you even find some of the flaws amusing or interesting. Maybe they give your friend color. Thinking about the flaws isn't likely to change your opinion or feelings, either.

Try applying the same perspective to yourself. Appreciate your little flaws, foibles, and quirks. They make you interesting and unique. Be a friend to yourself. Notice your gifts and your imperfections. Figure out how to acknowledge it all as one package. Don't disown your flaws.

TIP

Try this exercise we call "Appreciating Flawed Friends." You'll likely notice that you accept your friend, good and bad, positive or negative.

1. **In the notebook or file you have for exercises, make two columns.**

2. **Think of a good friend.**

3. **In the first column, write down a couple of the friend's positive qualities.**

4. **In the second column, describe a couple of negative qualities or imperfections that your friend has.**

Following this exercise, realize that your friends probably have a similar picture of you. The following example shows you how this particular exercise works for Curtis.

Curtis struggles with self-esteem and feels anxious about making mistakes or failing to be perfect. He tries filling out the "Appreciating Flawed Friends" exercise in Table 8-1 while thinking about his buddy Jack. In the respective columns, he writes about Jack's positive qualities and imperfections.

TABLE 8-1   **Appreciating Flawed Friends**

Positive Qualities	Negative Qualities and Imperfections
Jack is one of the funniest guys I know.	Sometimes Jack talks too much.
He's always there for me.	Even though he's smart, sometimes Jack makes stupid decisions, especially about money.
Jack will help me anytime I need it, no matter what.	Jack's a little overweight, and sometimes he drinks a little too much.
I like going to sporting events with him.	He doesn't always listen to me.
I like the fact that Jack is really smart.	Jack has terrible taste in clothes.

Curtis accepts Jack, flaws and all. There's no one that Curtis would rather spend time with, and Jack is the first person he would turn to in a crisis. Can Curtis accept himself like he does Jack? That's the task at hand.

If your friend filled out the same form on you, no doubt she would write about both wonderful qualities and some less-than-wonderful traits. And yet, your friend wouldn't suddenly give up the friendship because of your imperfections. Of course not; nobody's perfect. If we all gave up on our imperfect friends, we would have no friends at all.

Self-forgiveness is difficult. Perhaps even more difficult is finding out how to drop defensive barriers in response to criticism from others. Figure out how to listen to criticism. Consider the fact that it may at least have an element of truth. Appreciate that portion of truth.

Try acknowledging any sliver of truth that criticism contains. Perhaps it's true *sometimes*. Perhaps the criticism is partially applicable. Instead of putting up barriers to communication and problem-solving, admitting to some flaws brings people closer.

Finally, realize that neither you nor anyone you know is perfect. Accept the reality that we all have flaws. That's what makes us human and loveable!

Connecting with the Here and Now

In some ways, language represents the peak of evolutionary development. Language makes us human, gives us art, allows us to express complex ideas, and provides us with the tools for creating solutions to problems. At the same time, language lays the foundation for much of our emotional distress. How can that be?

You may think that dogs don't get anxious, but they do. However, they only feel anxiety when they're in direct contact with experiences that cause them pain or discomfort. For example, dogs rarely enjoy going to the vet. More than a few dog owners have had to drag their dogs through the veterinarian's door by pulling on the leash with all their might.

However, humans do what dogs would never do. Humans wake up dreading the events of the day that lies ahead. Dogs don't wake up at 3 a.m. and think, "Oh no! Is today the day that I have to go to the vet? What will happen to me there?"

And dogs have few regrets. Oh sure, sometimes dogs look pretty guilty when caught chewing on their master's shoe. But one kind word and a pat on the head, and they've forgotten all about it. Some anxious people still remember the thank-you note that they forgot to write to Aunt Betty six years ago.

Generally speaking, dogs seem much happier than most of us humans. Unless a dog has been horribly abused, he usually carries on with contentment, joy, and, of course, quite a bit of sleeping. By contrast, humans worry a lot; they obsess over imagined horrors down the road, and they dwell on their past mistakes.

When you bring possible future catastrophes as well as past regrets into the present, you're essentially using language to disconnect you from real-life experience. Doing so can absolutely ruin your *present moments* — the time that you actually *live* your entire life! Consider the following example of Reggie, who dreaded the amount of work that he believed he had to finish within five days.

> **Reggie,** a criminal defense attorney, has a solo practice. An important trial is coming up in five days. The amount of work in front of him almost chokes him with fear. Of course, he agonizes over the possibility of putting on a less-than-stellar performance, but most of all, he is concerned about the heavy preparation of papers, briefs, depositions, and petitions that must be completed — and soon. He knows that he'll be working from dawn to dusk with barely enough time to breathe.
>
> The funny thing about it, though, is that after the ordeal was over, he realized that most of those five days turned out to be fairly enjoyable. He worried over the possibility of not completing his tasks, which had nothing to do with any of the actual work that he performed. Most of that felt pretty good. Not a single, individual moment felt *horrible* by itself.

Few present moments truly feel unbearable. It's simply our ability to ruin the present with thoughts about the future or past that disturbs us.

The next time you obsess over future or past events, tasks, or outcomes, consider trying the following:

>> Stay focused on each moment as it comes to you.

>> Spend a few minutes noticing all the sensations in your body at the moment — touch, smell, sights, and sounds.

>> When thoughts about the tasks ahead enter your mind, simply acknowledge the presence of those thoughts, and move your attention back to the present.

>> If thoughts about past failures or regrets enter your mind, notice the presence of those thoughts, and move your attention back to the present.

>> Remind yourself that *thoughts* don't reflect reality and experience; they're only *thoughts*.

>> When you notice disturbing thoughts about the future or the past, try to just observe them, notice how interesting it is that your mind spins out thoughts like these, and return to the present moment.

The following sections contain specific exercises you can use to keep your mind focused on the present moment. We also offer some pointers on how to slow down and enjoy mealtimes and walks.

Making contact with the present

At this very moment, consider coming into direct contact with experience. This is something many people have rarely done. Have no expectations about what this exercise is *supposed* to do. Just study what happens.

If judgments enter your mind as you're doing the following exercise, observe how your mind spins these out like a reflex. Make no judgments about these thoughts or yourself. Go back to focusing on the entire array of present-moment sensations.

1. **Notice how this book feels in your hands.**

   Feel the smooth cover and the edges of the pages. Or feel the buttons and surface of your e-book reader!

2. **Notice how your body feels and notice your position, whether you're sitting, standing in a subway, riding a bus, or lying in bed.**

   Feel the sensations in your skin as it makes contact with the chair, the bed, the floor if you're standing, and so on.

3. **Feel the muscles in your legs, back, hands, and arms as you hold this book.**

4. **Notice your breathing.**

   Feel the air go in and out of your nostrils.

5. **Notice any smells, whether pleasant or unpleasant.**

   Think about how you could write a report about these smells.

6. **Listen to any sounds around you. Imagine how you would describe these sounds to a friend.**

   If you hear loud, obnoxious sounds, try *not* to judge them. Instead of thinking about how jarring they sound, study the nuances in the sounds.

Now, notice how you feel at the end of this exercise. Did you experience the sensations fully? What happened to your anxiety? Many people report that they feel little, if any, anxiety during this experience. Others say their anxiety escalates.

If your anxiety increases during your first few attempts to connect with present-moment experience, don't worry. It happens for various reasons. Increased anxiety doesn't mean that you're doing something wrong. More than likely, it can be attributed to one or more of the following:

>> You may have little experience connecting to the present. Therefore, it feels strange.

>> Anxious thoughts may interrupt you frequently. If so, more practice may help to reduce their potency.

>> You may be facing such an overwhelming stressor right now that putting this strategy into effect is unrealistic. If so, you may want to try other strategies in the book first.

Whatever the case, we recommend practicing frequent connection with present-moment experiences.

Most anxiety and distress come from thoughts about the future or the past, not what's happening at this moment.

REMEMBER

Putting worries about the future to rest

Most people tell us that at least 90 percent of what they worry about never happens. Of those worrisome events that do occur, less than 10 percent are as bad as they anticipated. That's an overabundance of worry and ruined present moments just to anticipate a few unpleasant occurrences.

Here's a way you can quit listening to that occasional stream of worries about future events.

TIP

1. **Think about how many times you've made negative forecasts in the past about some pending event.**

2. **Then, ask yourself how often those forecasts have proven true.**

   If you're not sure, keep a log of your negative predictions and see what percentage pans out.

3. **Of those forecasts that do come true, how often is it as bad as you anticipated?**

   If you're not sure how often, keep a log for a while.

Taking these predictions seriously is rather like listening to a weather reporter on the television who tells you that blizzards, severe cold, and ice storms are forecasted for every day. So, you dutifully don a heavy coat, gloves, and boots. Just one problem nags you, however. Ninety percent of the time, the reporter is absolutely wrong, and the weather is sunny and warm. When the reporter gets it almost right, rarely are conditions as bad as described. Perhaps it's time to stop listening to the weather reporter in your head. You can't turn the station off, but you can at least take the reports less seriously!

Being tolerant and flexible

Imagine you've been bitten by a mosquito. The itching is starting to drive you crazy! You want to scratch it, but you "know" better. So, you scratch around it. It's all you can think about. Okay, just one scratch — feels so good, but the itching increases. This is miserable, horrible, and will make your already boring night even worse. Glumly, you go to the refrigerator, open the door, and find nothing appealing. Ugh. You reach down and scratch that miserable mosquito bite again.

Your phone vibrates, signaling a text message. Your best friend wants to meet you for a walk. She's bored, too. You agree to meet in a half hour. You go to the bathroom, brush your hair, and grab a jacket. This will be a nice reprieve. After an enjoyable walk, you return home. You're watching the news, and you feel some itching return. Damn mosquito bite!

You realize that the whole time, from reading the text to just this second, you hadn't noticed your mosquito bite. You tolerated it and flexibly allowed yourself to engage with something more important. Ponder how you can use that tolerance and flexibility to deal with other minor irritations or itches in your life. Sometimes it's just a matter of paying attention to what's more important.

When you "can't stand" something, it inevitably overwhelms you. Flexible acceptance allows you to accept those small nuisances and become engaged with higher priorities in the present. Sometimes a little calamine lotion helps too!

Accepting Mindfulness into Your Life

Some people read about mindfulness and worry about the time it can consume. They say that it sounds like living life in slow motion and complain that nothing would ever get done if they tried living that way. As much as we think that living a little slower isn't a bad idea for many people, mindful acceptance doesn't require significant chunks of time.

More than time, mindfulness entails a shift in philosophy that decreases the focus on ego, pride, and control, while emphasizing accepting the present with all its gifts and challenges. Being mindful requires humility because it acknowledges the uncertainty that's inherent within life.

Making mindful acceptance a habit doesn't happen overnight. With practice, allow it to evolve slowly into your life. Accept that you won't always stay in the present. Don't judge your attempts to live mindfully. When you see yourself living in the guilt-ridden past or anxious future, gently remind yourself to come back to the present.

Savoring Spirituality

Accepting anxiety involves a variety of related attitudes, such as being nonjudgmental, tolerating uncertainty, letting go of the need for absolute control, and being patient. Realize that acceptance isn't the same as resignation or total surrender.

Acceptance means appreciating that you, as well as all humans, have strengths and limitations. Many people find that the process of acquiring acceptance leads them to a greater sense of spirituality — a feeling that the purpose of life transcends one's own self-concerns. *The Serenity Prayer* captures this spirit of acceptance nicely:

> *God, grant me the serenity*
>
> *to accept the things I cannot change,*
>
> *the courage to change the things I can,*
>
> *and the wisdom to know the difference.*
>
> *Living one day at a time;*
>
> *enjoying one moment at a time;*
>
> *accepting hardship as the pathway to peace.*
>
> *Taking, as He did, this sinful world as it is,*
>
> *not as I would have it.*
>
> *Trusting that He will make all things right*
>
> *if I surrender to His Will;*
>
> *that I may be reasonably happy in this life,*
>
> *and supremely happy with Him forever in the next.*
>
> *— Reinhold Niebuhr, 1926*

Chapter **9**

Facing Fear

When life hands you lemons, make lemonade. This advice sounds a lot easier to carry out than it is. Turning a situation around for the better after a series of hurts can be tough. Shifting to another metaphor, if you fall off your horse, everyone knows that it's best to jump right back into the saddle. But getting back up isn't always so easy to do either.

This chapter explains *how* you can get back in the saddle and even make some lemonade while you're up there (sorry). We show you how to overcome your fears in manageable steps. You don't have to face them all at once, because taking small steps does the trick. This chapter provides a recipe called *exposure* for overcoming your personal anxiety problem one step at a time.

But first, we want to convince you how avoiding bad feelings and things that make you anxious makes life much worse. It may seem counterintuitive, but the following sections will show you why avoidance is often thought to make a major contribution to the development and maintenance of anxiety.

All About Avoidance

Those who have no major problem with anxiety usually manage to cope fairly well with everyday stress. However, challenging circumstances, experiences, and even physical health problems alter and may reduce the ability to cope. When that happens, emotions that were relatively stable become shaky and unpleasant. So, a new coping strategy usually emerges. It's called *avoidance*. Initially, avoidance seems like a pretty reasonable way to work around new, uncomfortable feelings.

However, avoidance, like a wickedly malignant virus, attacks healthy behaviors and destroys your efforts to feel better. The vast majority of people would choose not to feel anxious if they could. In fact, part of your motivation to buy this book may have been to figure out how to reduce such unpleasant feelings. Just one problem: Avoidance does nothing but make things worse. A lot worse. The following sections discuss what people avoid, how they avoid it, and why avoidance doesn't work.

REMEMBER

Research has repeatedly shown that people who try to avoid unpleasant thoughts, memories, emotions, and experiences actually suffer more emotional distress, especially anxiety.

TIP

Avoidance almost always feels good in the short run. But, over time, it rarely pays off. Your willingness to suffer some anxiety in the present will paradoxically reduce your anxiety down the road.

Avoiding emotions

No one wants to feel bad. When you are about to go into a stressful meeting or interview, or give a presentation, have you ever said to yourself, "Calm down, stop being so nervous"? Does telling yourself to stop feeling anxious reliably work for you? Most people find it doesn't. In fact, when people fail to calm down, they usually feel more anxiety than if they'd done nothing at all.

Emotional avoidance involves an attempt to suppress unwanted feelings, hoping they'll go away. Usually emotional avoidance represents an attempt to eliminate negative emotions such as anxiety, fear, panic, or even depression.

TIP

Occasionally, a brief avoidance of emotions makes sense, such as during an emergency. For example, if your child falls into a lake, you would probably put your fear of the water aside to attempt a rescue. Firefighters run into burning buildings despite knowing the danger. At times of great crises, it can be an adaptive strategy to become numb while you figure out what to do.

TECHNICAL STUFF

A few people with anxiety actually try to avoid positive emotions like calm and serene. Why? Because when they feel calm, they believe that those feelings will result in letting their guard down. When their guard is down, they report feeling more vulnerable. So, they surprisingly try to engineer an uptick in fear and anxiety to defend against an anticipated attack.

Obvious avoidance of what you fear

Anxious people don't simply try to avoid unpleasant feelings, they also engage in avoidant behaviors. That means doing everything and anything they can to avoid situations and events that have the potential to cause anxiety. For example:

>> Someone who's afraid of elevators consistently takes the stairs.

>> A person who fears public speaking takes a job in data entry.

>> A socially anxious person avoids parties or large groups even when there isn't a pandemic going on.

>> Someone who experiences panic in theaters doesn't go to movies or plays.

>> Someone who fears being trapped in public stays at home.

TIP

Like emotional avoidance, engaging in obvious avoidant behavior actually manages to increase rather than decrease fear.

More subtle avoidance strategies

It's pretty easy to spot avoidance when someone takes the stairs to avoid the elevator or someone with a dog phobia stays out of dog parks. However, there are many subtle forms of avoidance. Some of the most common strategies for subtly sidestepping anxiety include

>> Not even trying to succeed due to worry about failure

>> Dressing down to avoid attention

>> Carrying a good luck charm to ward off harm

>> Carrying anxiety medication, "just in case"

>> Avoiding checkups and doctors to keep from hearing bad news

>> Always arriving exactly on time to avoid criticism

>> Avoiding situations that trigger bad memories

>> Tuning out and distracting yourself from anxious feelings

>> Avoiding conflict at all cost

>> Tamping down feelings to avoid feeling pain

>> Numbing via drugs, alcohol, or overeating

>> Scrolling through a cellphone to avoid interacting with people

>> Engaging in rituals such as repeating a series of numbers or slogans

>> Napping to disengage

>> Looking for distractions of almost any kind

>> Avoiding feelings associated with panic by avoiding things like exercise or hot rooms

Whether you arrive late and leave early or pretend to be immersed in fascinating messages on your phone, these are simply ways to avoid social interaction. Avoidance ends up making you more nervous and intolerant of anxiety. Other people may not even have a clue that you're nervous or that you're doing all you can to reduce your anxiety. Indeed, they may think nothing at all or that you're rude. But the bottom line is that almost all avoidance strategies — whether subtle or obvious — backfire. They make your anxiety worse.

Breaking the avoidance cycle

Why does avoidance make anxiety worse? If you're nervous about something, and you stay away from it, you feel great relief. Let's face it; relief feels really good. You don't have to deal with something that makes you feel anxious and afraid. Congratulations, you've rewarded yourself by avoiding those bad feelings. Just one problem: The next time something anxiety-arousing comes along, you're likely to do the same. Avoidance takes root and grows.

Here's an example of how the avoidance cycle works.

Amihan has three school-aged children. She's from the Philippines and has lived in the United States for over a decade. She can't seem to shake her intense shyness and anxiety in social situations. Her husband (a physician who works nights) usually attends the children's events like parent-teacher conferences and school bake sales.

Every time he helps his wife avoid a social or kid-oriented event, she feels a lot of gratitude and relief. She also notices that her social anxiety has been increasing slowly over time. She used to at least walk her kids to the bus stop and talk to a few of the parents. Lately, she's been avoiding even that.

Here's how Amihan's avoidance cycle works:

1. She contemplates going to a school open house but experiences intense social anxiety. Just thinking about it makes her stomach ache, her hands sweat, and she feels short of breath.

2. She tells her husband that she doesn't feel good. So, she decides to stay home and asks him to attend. He reluctantly agrees.

3. She immediately feels a powerful surge of relief.

4. The next time a similar event comes up, she repeats the cycle.

If Amihan doesn't find a way to break the avoidance cycle, her anxiety will merely deepen and spread to other similar events. Eventually, it could cause problems with her entire family.

TIP

The avoidance cycle is surprisingly powerful. Even people who don't have major problems with anxiety sometimes fall into the seductive trap of avoiding what feels bad in the short run. Procrastination is a common example of avoiding an unpleasant task. It makes you feel better in the short run. But it bangs you in the back of the head eventually.

Accepting discomfort and distress

If you spend much of your life trying to avoid discomfort and distress, you're likely to find yourself stymied and missing out on countless opportunities, challenges, joys, and excitement. For example, a novice skier who doesn't progress after mastering the bunny hill will never feel the excitement of mastering a more difficult slope. A promising student who fears failure may not complete her thesis — better not to try than to try and fail. If she continues this pattern, she'll never experience the joy of accomplishing her life's dreams.

TIP

Anxiety will only deepen and intensify if you're not willing to *accept* a certain amount of discomfort and distress. The following pointers show you the steps for how to start accepting a little angst in your life.

1. Pause.

When you feel discomfort, stop; don't run. Don't make an immediate decision on what to do next. Sit with your uneasiness a while. Take a few breaths. Find a different perspective. Instead of thinking how awful you feel, notice and observe. Prepare to do something different this time.

2. Assess.

Ask yourself what you're feeling anxious about. Now, what is your anxiety telling you to do or not to do? What are your options? What's likely to happen depending on which option you choose? What's the worst that could happen to you if you take one option versus the other? How much discomfort are you willing to take on?

3. Act.

Once you've paused and assessed your situation, pick the option that looks best to you. That doesn't mean take the option that will make you feel best;

rather, choose the one that feels like an accomplishment and a step forward. Your selection doesn't have to be massive — just do something! If your choice doesn't get you what you hoped it would, that's something to learn from and accept. Every action moves you ahead.

The previous pointers pave the way for the tougher tasks that lie ahead in the following sections.

Exposure: Coming to Grips with Your Fears

No single strategy discussed in this book works more effectively in the fight against anxiety than exposure. Simply put, exposure involves putting yourself in direct contact with whatever it is that makes you anxious. Well now, that may just sound a little ridiculous to you.

After all, it probably makes you feel pretty anxious to even think about staring your fears in the face. We understand that reaction, but please realize that if you're terrified of heights, exposure doesn't ask you to lean over the edge of the Grand Canyon tomorrow. Or, if you worry about having a panic attack in crowds, you don't have to sit in the stands of the next Super Bowl as your first step.

Exposure involves a systematic, gradual set of steps that you tackle one at a time. You'll probably want to start with an exposure that doesn't push you over the edge — something modestly difficult will do just fine. You don't necessarily move from that initial first step until you master it, but it's fine if you want to try. When you're reasonably comfortable with the first step, you move to the second, or if you're up to it, the third. Each new step will likely bring on more anxiety, but not an overwhelming amount.

The following sections show you how to create an exposure plan for your own fear. For example, a person who fears leaving home would develop a plan to first walk to the mailbox and then around the block before going farther from home. Similarly, someone who fears driving on the freeway would probably choose a plan that starts with multilane but uncrowded streets, then busy streets followed by driving on an uncrowded freeway on an early Sunday morning. The plan would advance in difficulty as each step is managed. Exposures are always individualized and go at a pace that works for each person.

TIP

If you find yourself procrastinating with the recommendations in this chapter, read Chapter 4 to build motivation and overcome obstacles to change. If you still find these ideas difficult to consider, you probably want to consult a professional for help.

Don't try exposure if your anxiety is severe. You'll need professional guidance. If any step raises your anxiety to an extreme level, stop any further attempt without help. Also, don't attempt exposure if you're in the midst of a crisis or have a current problem with alcohol or substance abuse — get help for those issues first.

Understanding your fears

Breaking up the exposure process into manageable steps is important. But before you can break your fears into steps, it helps to fully understand the nature of what makes you fearful. Try the following strategies:

1. **Pick one of your worries.**

    For example, you might be afraid of one of the following:

    -   Enclosed spaces

    -   Financial ruin

    -   Flying

    -   Excessive worry about the well-being of loved ones

    -   Having a panic attack (a fear of a fear)

    -   Social events

2. **Think about every conceivable aspect of your fear or worry.**

    What starts up your fear? Include all the activities that surround it. For example, if you're afraid of flying, perhaps you fear driving to the airport or packing your luggage. Or if you're afraid of dogs, you may avoid walking near them, and you probably don't visit people who have dogs. Wherever the fear starts, take some notes on it. Think about all the anticipated and feared outcomes. What are you thinking; how are you feeling? Include all the details, like other people's reactions and the setting.

3. **Ask yourself the following questions and jot down your answers:**

    -   How does my anxiety begin?

    -   What activities do I avoid?

    -   Do I use any subtle avoidance strategies?

    -   Do I use alcohol, medications, or other drugs to numb my anxiety?

    -   What are all the things I'd have to do if I actually faced my fear head-on?

    -   What other situations are affected by my fear?

    -   Do I use any crutches to get through my fear? If so, what are they?

    -   What bad outcomes do I anticipate if I were to encounter my fear?

TIP

Using the question–answer format, you can describe what you're afraid of. Use your imagination. Don't let embarrassment keep you from including the deepest, darkest aspects of your fears, even if you think they may sound silly to someone else.

Leeann's story is a good illustration of how someone completes this exercise to enrich her understanding of her fears.

Leeann, a 32-year-old pharmaceutical representative, receives a promotion, which means a large increase in salary and plenty of air travel. During her interview, Leeann doesn't mention her intense fear of flying, somehow hoping that it will just go away. Now, in three weeks she faces her first flight, and her distress prompts her to seek help.

She reads about exposure and concludes that it's the best approach for her problem. To see how Leeann completes the first task — understanding her fear and all its components — see Table 9-1.

TABLE 9-1 **What I'm Afraid Of**

Question	Answer
How does my anxiety begin?	The very thought of flying makes me anxious. Even driving on the same road that leads to the airport gets me worked up.
What activities do I avoid?	I've avoided vacations and trips with friends and family in order to avoid flying.
Do I use any subtle avoidance?	Yes, I pretend that I don't really like traveling to avoid it.
Do I use drugs or alcohol to numb?	Sometimes I do, but not usually.
What are all the things I'd have to do if I actually faced my fear head-on?	I'd have to make a reservation. Then, I'd have to pack my luggage, drive to the airport, go through security, spend some time in the waiting area, hear my flight called, and board the plane. Then I'd take a seat and go through takeoff. Finally, I'd endure the flight.
What other situations are affected by my fear?	If I don't get over this, I'll never get my promotion at work. Not only that, I'll continue to feel embarrassed around friends and family whenever the topic comes up.
Do I use crutches to get through my fear? If so, what are they?	One time I got on an airplane and got sick to my stomach because I'd had too much to drink in order to calm my nerves.
What bad outcomes do I anticipate if I were to encounter my fear?	I fear that I'd go crazy, throw up on the passengers next to me, or start screaming, and they'd have to restrain me. Of course, the plane could crash, and then I'd die or suffer horrible burns and pain, unable to get out of the plane.

You can see that Leeann's fear of flying consists of several activities, from making a reservation to getting off the plane. Her anticipated outcomes include a range of what she considers to be unpleasant possibilities.

Constructing an exposure list

The preceding section helps you comprehend the nature of your fears. After you come to that understanding, you're ready to take your fear apart, and construct a list of exposure goals. Here's how to do it:

1. **Make a list of each and every single thing you'd have to do if you were to ultimately, totally face your fear.**

   Consider including a few items that you may want to do in anticipation of facing your ultimate fear (such as looking at pictures of what you fear, imagining yourself in the feared situation, or talking with other people about your fear).

2. **Rate each one on a scale of 0 to 10.**

   Zero represents the total absence of fear, and 10 indicates a fear that's unimaginably intense and totally debilitating.

3. **Arrange the items into a list beginning with the lowest-rated item at the bottom and ending with the most difficult item on the top.**

   This constitutes your exposure hierarchy. Just making your list may cause you some anxiety. Again, don't worry; you will most likely choose to approach each step one at a time. Besides, the goal isn't to avoid all anxiety; you actually *want* to invite anxiety into your life, and allow it to stay a while. You just may discover it's not as terrifying as you thought.

Leeann has a phobia about flying. (See the earlier section "Understanding your fears.") She lists the following steps that all directly lead to her ultimate fear — flying by herself. She starts with relatively "easy" items and then moves toward more difficult goals. Again, the point is not to avoid all anxiety, but to embrace modest levels.

» Visit an airport without flying (3)

» Read about airplane safety and crashes (3)

» Talk to people about travel plans (3)

» Talk to ten people about their worst experiences flying (4)

» Get some travel brochures and search online for information (4)

>> Watch videos of airplane crashes (6)

>> Make a reservation for an air flight (8)

>> Go on a short flight with a friend (9)

>> Go on a longer trip by myself (10)

So, now you have seen an example of an exposure list. If you haven't tried making one, do so now — it can focus on airplanes or any other fear you may have. Select a fear or a group of worries with a similar theme. For example, fear of rejection is a theme that involves lots of worries about criticism and evaluation by others. Similarly, anxiety about personal injury is a theme that involves a variety of fears about safety. Break the fear into a number of sequential steps, with each step being slightly more difficult than the prior step. If you need more help, we give more examples throughout this chapter.

Facing your fears (gulp)

Once you've made your list, it's time to face your fears head-on. First, select an item from your exposure list that looks doable to you. Table 9-2 shows you how Leeann, with her fear of flying, began her first exposure and carried out our suggested directions for exposure. You can do the same.

TABLE 9-2 **Leeann's Exposure Procedures**

Directions	Response
Write down my chosen exposure task.	Visit the airport.
Thoughts I had before actually starting the exposure.	This doesn't seem too hard. But I usually get nervous when the airport gets close. I hate getting anxious.
From 0 to 10, how hard do I think this will be?	I think it will be a 3.
Do the task.	I drove to the airport and went inside.
Rate how hard the task was on a scale of 0–10.	I'd give it a 6. It was harder than I thought it would be.
Jot down my thoughts, feelings, and behaviors during my exposure.	I gripped the steering wheel really hard and felt sweaty and tense. When I went into the airport, my stomach flipped.
My thoughts, feelings, and behaviors after completing the task.	Wow. I think I realized that I was on a journey to conquer my fear. That made me both proud and frightened. I guess a little fear is okay. I'm ready to tackle the next item on my exposure list!

After you've completed your first exposure goal, plan when and how you want to tackle your next item. Keep on going until you're able to get over the goal line consistently.

The following hints can help you get through the exposure process:

» Don't let lots of time go by without taking on another exposure item. For some people, once a week is enough, but that's on the low end. Taking on an item every day is not excessive if you have the time and it feels okay to you.

» Enlist the help of an exposure buddy, but only if you have someone you really trust. This person can give you encouragement and support. Only use a buddy in the early exposure stages. You want to learn how to master exposure on your own eventually.

» If you must, back off your step just a little. Don't make a complete retreat unless you feel absolutely out of control.

» Your mind will tell you, "Stop! You can't do this. It won't work anyway." Don't listen to this chatter. Simply study your body's reactions, as well as your behaviors and thoughts. Realize that these reactions, behaviors, and thoughts are good for you! You will learn from them.

» Find a way to reward yourself for each successful step you take. Perhaps indulge in a desired purchase or treat yourself in some other way. For example, you could put a few bucks in a shoebox each time you complete a step, with a goal of rewarding yourself with a larger treat after you've made substantial progress.

» Understand that at times, you will feel uncomfortable. View that discomfort as progress; it's part of how you overcome your fears.

» Practice, practice, practice.

» Remember to stay with each step as your anxiety drops a little. Realize that your body can't maintain anxiety forever. It's likely to come down if you give it some time. But it's actually helpful to experience and be in touch with a reasonable degree of anxiety. Accept that emotion as part of being a human being.

» Don't expect an instant cure. Proceed at a reasonable pace. Keep moving forward, but don't expect to conquer your fear in a few days. Even with daily practice, exposure can take a number of months.

Remember to set realistic goals. For example, say you're afraid of spiders — so much so that you can't enter a room without an exhaustive search for hidden horrors. You don't have to perform exposure exercises to the point where you let tarantulas crawl up and down your arms. Let yourself feel satisfied with the ability to enter rooms without unnecessary checking.

WARNING

Try to avoid using crutches to avoid fully exposing yourself to your exposure list. Some of the popular crutches that people use include the following:

>> Drinking alcohol

>> Taking tranquilizers, especially the benzodiazepines we discuss in Chapter 10

>> Distracting themselves with rituals, song lyrics, or chants

>> Holding onto something to keep from fainting

>> Asking someone else to reassure them that everything will be okay if they carry out an exposure item

All of these crutches actually interfere with the effectiveness of exposure. But if you absolutely feel the need to use one of these crutches, use as little as you can. Furthermore, don't hold onto crutches for very long — they get in the way. Walk your own walk.

Conquering Different Types of Fears

Confronting your fears directly is one of the most powerful ways of overcoming them. But your exposure plan can look different, depending on the particular type of anxiety you have. This section lays out example plans for some of the most common types of anxiety. You'll no doubt need to individualize these for dealing with your problem. However, they should help you get started.

TIP

You can find more examples of exposure lists by searching online for "examples of anxiety exposure hierarchies."

Waging war on worry

Some people worry about most everything. As a result of that worry, they usually end up avoiding a variety of opportunities and other tasks of everyday life. These worries can rob their victims of pleasure and enjoyment.

Chloe's story shows you how someone with worrisome amounts of worry tackles some of her fears.

> **Chloe's** friends call her a worrywart, and her children call her "the prison guard." Chloe frets constantly, but her biggest worry is the safety of her 16-year-old twin boys. Unfortunately, Chloe's worry causes her to restrict her kids' activities far more than most parents do. She doesn't allow them out of the house after dark, so they

can't participate in extracurricular activities. Chloe interrogates them about every new friend. As the kids get older, they rebel. Squabbles and fights dominate dinner, but the biggest bone of contention revolves around learning to drive. Although both are eligible to take driver's education, Chloe declares that they can't drive until they're at least 18 years old.

Chloe is surprised when the school counselor calls her to discuss her sons' concerns. He meets with her for a few sessions and helps Chloe to realize that her worries are overblown. She knows she has a problem and decides to tackle it head-on.

After helping her understand that her worries are over the top, the counselor suggests that Chloe talk to other parents at her church to get a reality check. She finds out that most parents allow their 16-year-old kids to attend supervised evening activities, to take driver's education, and even drive if they maintain good grades.

Chloe constructs her exposure list, starting from the least fearful item to the most terrifying. She rates the difficulty from low (1) to high (10). Here's what she comes up with:

>> Drop my sons off to attend a sports event by themselves (3)

>> Allow my sons to go to a school dance unaccompanied (3)

>> Sign up the kids for driver's education (5)

>> Let the boys practice driving with their dad (6)

>> Practice driving by myself with the boys (8)

>> Let my sons take a driver's test (8)

>> Allow the kids to drive to a nearby friend's house on their own (9)

After Chloe comes up with her exposure list, she's ready to get to work. She picks the first task and completes the exposure directions in Table 9-3.

If you have excessive worry, pick one of your various troubling concerns. Then, construct your personal exposure list to address that particular worry. Once you have your list, start with a fairly easy task and expose yourself.

REMEMBER

Construct your list with enough items so that you will have multiple opportunities to experience increasing levels of difficulty. Complete exposure procedures for each item on your list. If you find one step insurmountable, try coming up with an in-between step. If you can't do that, try taking the tough step through repeated imaginary exposures before tackling it in real life. And, as always, don't hesitate to get professional help if exposure feels like too much.

TABLE 9-3   **Chloe's Exposure Procedures**

Directions	Response
Write down my chosen exposure task.	I dropped my sons off to attend a sports event by themselves.
Thoughts I had before actually starting the exposure.	Are they going to be okay? I don't know what I'd do if they got hurt. Other kids could talk them into being reckless!
From 0 to 10, how hard do I think this will be?	Initially, it seemed like this would be a 2 or a 3. But now, I'm afraid it's a 9. I'll give it a go anyway.
Do the task.	I did it! They went to a football game by themselves and survived.
Rate how hard the task was on a scale of 0–10.	I'd give it a 5.
Jot down my thoughts, feelings, and behaviors during my exposure.	I was a bit worried, more so when I first dropped them off, but I settled down. My heart raced a little for a few minutes, and I drove around the block a few times.
My thoughts, feelings, and behaviors after completing the task.	I can see where this is really good for me to do. The boys need to become more independent. I can do this.

Fighting phobias

You fight phobias of all kinds in pretty much the same way. Take the feared situation, object, animal, people, or whatever, and approach it in graduated steps. Again, you construct an exposure list consisting of a series of small steps. Ruben's story is a good example of how an exposure list helped someone with a phobia — in this case, a fear of heights.

> **Ruben** meets Diane through a dating app. They text back and forth for several weeks. Finally, they decide to meet for coffee. Several hours pass in what seems like minutes to both of them, and Ruben offers to walk Diane home.
>
> As he holds the restaurant door open for her, her body brushes against him. Their eyes meet, and Ruben almost kisses her right there in the doorway. As they walk toward her apartment building, she asks, "Do you believe in love at first sight?" Ruben doesn't hesitate. "Yes," he answers, wrapping her in his arms. The kiss is so intense that Ruben thinks he might collapse on the spot.
>
> "I've never done this before on a first date, but I think I'd like you to come up to my place," Diane says, as she strokes his arm. "I have a wonderful view of the entire city from my penthouse apartment."
>
> Ruben looks up at the 25-story apartment building. His desire shrinks. "Ah, well, I've got to pick up Mom, I mean the cat at the vet," he stammers. Diane, obviously hurt and surprised, snaps, "Fine. I've really got to wash my socks."

Ruben decides to fight his phobia. He constructs an exposure list out of steps that start at the bottom and go all the way to the most fearful step at the top.

Confessing his problem to Diane is a step that may appear unrelated to Ruben's fear. However, not admitting to his fear is avoidance, which only fuels fear. Including any step that's connected to your fear is good. Ruben also included steps in his list that required him to use his imagination to face his fear. It's fine to do that. Sometimes, imaginary steps can help you take the next behavioral step. The following list starts with relatively easy items and ends with the most difficult. Ruben thinks that getting to Diane's penthouse will be worth the struggle.

>> Calling Diane and telling her about my phobia and that I'd really like to see her again (4)

>> Imagining going up the elevator to visit with Diane in her penthouse (4)

>> Walking across a pedestrian bridge that has a fence around it (5)

>> Walking up three flights of stairs and peering down (6)

>> Taking a glass elevator with Diane at a downtown hotel and looking out over the city (7)

>> Doing the same thing by myself (8)

>> Visiting Diane in her penthouse apartment and seeing what happens (10)

REMEMBER

Imagining the real-life steps before actually doing them doesn't hurt and will likely help prepare you for the real thing. And don't forget, it's okay to try something with a buddy as long as you do it on your own later.

Pushing through panic

Some people experience periods of time that they label as panic. A panic attack usually involves rushes of adrenaline, a racing heart, shortness of breath, and a feeling of dread or doom. (See Chapter 2 for more information about panic attacks.) Tanya's story depicts how someone who experiences panic attacks develops an exposure list.

Tanya experiences her first panic attack shortly after the birth of her baby. Always somewhat shy, she begins to worry about something happening to herself when she takes the baby out. She fears that she might faint or lose control, leaving the baby vulnerable to harm.

Her panic attacks start with a feeling of nervousness and sweaty palms, and then progress to shallow, rapid breathing, a racing heartbeat, lightheadedness, and a sense of dread and doom. Trips away from the house trigger her attacks, and the more crowded the destination, the more likely she is to experience panic. By six months after her first attack, she rarely leaves the house without her husband.

One day, Tanya's baby girl develops a serious fever, and she needs to take her to the emergency room. Panic overtakes her; she frantically calls her husband, but he's out on a business call. Desperate, she calls 911 to send an ambulance.

Tanya knows that she must do something about her panic disorder. She constructs an exposure list out of a set of steps, starting with the least problematic and progressing to the most difficult goal.

Tanya needs to make each step very gradual to have the courage to proceed. She could make the steps even smaller, if necessary. Here's are a few of the items she conjured up for her exposure tasks:

>> I'll put the baby in a stroller and walk around the block (2)

>> I'll take the baby to my mother's house, which is five miles away (3)

>> I'll take the baby on an errand (5)

>> I'll take the baby to the pediatrician by myself (7)

>> I'll leave the baby with my husband and go grocery shopping by myself (8)

REMEMBER

You can break your staircase of fear down into as many small steps as you need to avoid feeling overwhelmed by taking any single step. But taking somewhat larger steps is just fine as well; it's your choice.

Another type of exposure that aims specifically at panic attacks involves experiencing the sensations of the attacks themselves. How do you do that? You repeatedly and intentionally bring them on through a number of strategies, as follows:

>> **Running in place:** This accelerates your heartbeat, just as many panic attacks do. Run for at least three to five minutes.

>> **Spinning yourself around until you feel dizzy:** Panic attacks often include sensations of dizziness and lightheadedness.

>> **Breathing through a small cocktail straw:** This strategy induces sensations of not getting enough air, which also mimics panic. Try this for a good 60 seconds at a time.

>> **Putting your head between your knees and rising up suddenly:** You may feel lightheaded or dizzy.

After you experience these physical sensations repeatedly, you discover that they don't harm you. You won't go crazy, have a heart attack, or lose control. Frequent, prolonged exposures tell your mind that sensations are just sensations.

WARNING

Don't bring on these physical sensations if you have a serious heart condition or any other physical problem that could be exacerbated by the exercise. For example, if you have asthma or a back injury, some of these strategies are ill-advised. Check with your doctor if you have any questions or concerns.

Expecting the Impossible

Occasionally, people have come to us asking for a quick fix for their anxiety problems. It's as though they thought we had some magic wand we could pass over them to make everything better. That would be so nice, but it isn't realistic.

Other folks hope that with help, they'll rid themselves of all anxiety — another misconception. Some anxiety helps prepare you for action, warn you of danger, and mobilize your resources (see Chapter 3).

The only people who are completely rid of anxiety are unconscious or dead.

REMEMBER

Overcoming anxiety requires effort and some discomfort. We have no way around that. No magic wand. But we know that those who undertake the challenge, make the effort, and suffer the discomfort are rewarded with reduced anxiety and increased confidence.

Chapter **10**

Medications and Other Biological Options

The last several decades have witnessed an explosion in new knowledge about emotions, mental illness, and brain chemistry. Scientists recognize changes in the brain that accompany many psychological disorders. New and old drugs attempt to address these chemical imbalances, and using these drugs has both advantages and disadvantages. Nonetheless, you should know that today, most mental health professionals view psychotherapy as the treatment of choice for a large majority of those who suffer from excessive anxiety.

This chapter helps you make an informed decision about whether or not to use medication for your anxiety. We give you information about the most widely pre-scribed classes of drugs and some of their more common side effects. Only you, in consultation with your healthcare provider, can determine what's best for helping you. Next, we tell you about over-the-counter supplements for anxiety. More importantly, we share the latest information about their effectiveness and warn you about possible dangers and downsides. Finally, we alert you to some of the methods that involve stimulating the brain for those whose anxiety is severe and resistant to standard treatments.

Making Up Your Mind About Medications

Deciding whether to medicate your anxiety brings up a number of issues to consider. This decision isn't one to take lightly. You should consult with your therapist, if you have one, as well as your physician. Before you decide on medication, ask yourself what you've done to alleviate your anxiety. Have you challenged your anxious thoughts and beliefs (see Chapters 5, 6, and 7)? Have you tried mindfully accepting your anxiety (see Chapter 8)? Have you faced your fears head-on (see Chapter 9)?

TIP

With a few important exceptions, which we review in this chapter, we recommend that you try various psychological approaches prior to adding medication. Why? Consider the following:

>> Medications only target symptoms, whereas psychotherapy takes a holistic approach. Psychotherapy contributes to growth, coping, and independence.

>> Some research suggests that certain medications may actually interfere with the long-term effectiveness of the most successful treatments for anxiety. That's especially true of the techniques designed to confront phobias and fears directly through exposure.

>> If you try psychological strategies first, you very well may discover that you don't need medication. Many of our recommended anxiety axes have the potential to cement change for the long haul as well as positively affect your entire life.

>> Studies show that variations of cognitive behavioral therapy (the type of strategies we discuss throughout this book) help prevent relapse. Many people who take medication alone experience a quick reoccurrence of symptoms when they discontinue taking medication for any reason.

The downside of medications

You need to reflect on both sides of any important decision. Medications have an upside and a downside. The negative side of the argument includes the following considerations:

>> **Addiction:** Some medications can lead to physical and/or mental dependency. Getting off of those medications can be difficult, or even dangerous, if not done properly. (However, contrary to what some people think, many medications are available that do *not* have addictive potential.)

>> **Long-term effects:** Some medications can lead to serious problems, such as diabetes and tremors.

>> **Philosophical aversions:** Some people just feel strongly that they don't like to take medications. And that's okay, but only to a point.

>> **Pregnancy and breast-feeding:** Only a few drugs are recommended for women who are pregnant or breast-feeding. The potential effects on the baby or fetus are just too risky for most situations.

>> **Side effects:** Most medications have various side effects, such as gastrointestinal upset, headaches, dizziness, dry mouth, and sexual dysfunction. Working with your physician to find the right medication — a drug that alleviates your anxiety and doesn't cause you overly troublesome side effects — may take some time.

The upside of medications

Sometimes medications make good sense. In weighing the pros and cons, we suggest that you take a good look at the benefits that medications can offer:

>> When serious depression accompanies anxiety, medication can sometimes provide faster relief, especially when a person feels hopeless, helpless, or suicidal.

>> Some people can't benefit from psychotherapy because of lack of access due to limited health insurance. In the short run, medications are usually cheaper.

>> Some people have impaired cognitive capacity that may limit their ability to benefit from psychotherapy (although there are modifications that can often be made).

>> When anxiety severely interferes with your life, medication sometimes provides relief more quickly than therapy or lifestyle changes. Such interferences include

- Panic attacks that occur frequently and cause expensive trips to the emergency room.

- Anxiety that feels so severe that you stop going to work or miss out on important life events.

>> When you've tried the recommendations in this book, consulted a qualified therapist, and you still suffer from excessive anxiety, medication may provide relief.

» If your physician tells you that your stress level must be controlled quickly to control your high blood pressure, that blood pressure medication may, in a few cases, also reduce your stress, in addition to adding a few years to your life.

» When you experience a sudden, traumatic event, a brief regimen of the right medication may help you get through it. When using medication for trauma, one should keep its use limited in duration to avoid dependency. Traumas, at least one of which happens to most people at one time or another include

- The sudden death of a loved one

- An unexpected accident

- Severe illness

- An unexpected financial disaster

- A natural disaster, such as a hurricane or earthquake

- Being the victim of a serious crime

- Being the victim of terrorism

TECHNICAL STUFF

In addition to an uptick of anxiety, trauma sometimes leads to a condition known as *post-traumatic stress disorder* (PTSD). PTSD is a serious condition that requires specialized psychological treatment and sometimes medication. However, PTSD is no longer considered an anxiety disorder even though anxiety usually forms part of the picture.

Understanding Medication Options

Today, physicians have a wide range of medications for the treatment of anxiety disorders. New drugs and applications appear all the time. Our list provides a brief overview of the major types of medications used for anxiety-related problems. We don't discuss each specific medication because new ones are being added all the time and differences among them can be dizzying. Our review is not intended to replace professional medical advice.

WARNING

If you decide to ask your doctor about medication, don't forget to discuss the following critical issues if they apply to you. Communicating with your doctor about these considerations can help prevent a bad outcome. Be sure to tell your doctor if you

» Are pregnant or plan to become pregnant

» Are breast-feeding

>> Drink alcohol

>> Take any other prescription drugs

>> Take any over-the-counter medications

>> Take herbs or supplements

>> Have any serious medical conditions

>> Have had any bad reactions to medications in the past

>> Have any allergies

>> Take birth control pills (some medications for anxiety reduce their effectiveness)

Most drugs prescribed for anxiety belong to one of the following categories:

>> Antidepressants

>> Benzodiazepines (minor tranquilizers)

>> Miscellaneous tranquilizers

>> Beta blockers

>> Atypical antipsychotics

>> Mood stabilizers

You may notice that some of these categories sound a little strange. For example, antidepressants (typically used to treat depression) and beta blockers (generally prescribed for hypertension) don't sound like groups of medications for the treatment of anxiety. But we show you that they play an important role with certain types of anxiety.

Antidepressants

Antidepressant medications have been used to treat anxiety for many decades. That's interesting because anxiety and depression often occur together. And both problems appear to have some similarity in terms of their biological underpinnings. Antidepressants increase the availability of different neurotransmitters or chemical messengers in the brain. The most frequently prescribed antidepressants increase the levels of serotonin, which helps regulate mood, anxiety, and the ability to control impulses.

Selective serotonin reuptake inhibitors (SSRIs)

Doctors prescribe SSRIs for all types of anxiety disorders. The SSRIs increase levels of the critical neurotransmitter serotonin at the nerve synapses by inhibiting the reabsorption of serotonin into the nerve cells. Serotonin helps stabilize mood. You should know that SSRIs still have significant side effects, though they tend to be milder than earlier types of antidepressants, and some ease with time.

WARNING

Side effects from SSRIs can include sedation, stomach upset, headaches, dizziness, weight gain, insomnia, restlessness, irritability, sexual problems, unusual behaviors, and even thoughts of suicide. Talk to your prescribing professional about any and all side effects. And get help immediately if you feel suicidal.

WARNING

SSRIs can interact with other drugs and, in rare cases, can cause life-threatening interactions. Be sure to tell your doctor about all medications or over-the-counter supplements you're taking.

Designer antidepressants

This class of antidepressants targets serotonin and other neurotransmitters, especially norepinephrine, that have different effects than the more commonly prescribed SSRIs. Some of these neurotransmitters boost energy and alertness while others affect experiences of pleasure, motivation, and attention. Common side effects of various antidepressant designer medications include increased sedation, insomnia, nausea, and anxiety.

Tricyclic antidepressants

Doctors usually try to treat anxiety with the newer antidepressant medications discussed in the previous two sections. However, when those medications don't do the trick, sometimes the tricyclic antidepressants work. Tricyclic antidepressants can take anywhere from two to twelve weeks to exert maximum effectiveness.

WARNING

Some people temporarily experience *increased* anxiety with tricyclic medications. In large part due to side effects that can increase anxiety and agitation, nearly 30 percent of patients discontinue taking tricyclic antidepressants.

That's why many physicians prescribe medication for anxiety disorders by starting with a low dosage and slowly increasing it as necessary. In other words, they prescribe a very low dose initially in order for your body to adjust to it with minimal side effects. They gradually increase the dosage in order to minimize negative reactions. It can take a while to reach an effective dose this way, but you'll probably find yourself able to tolerate the medication more easily.

Even with careful dosing, tricyclic medications can cause considerable side effects, including dizziness, weight gain, dry mouth, blurred vision, and constipation. Some of these effects resolve over time, but many of them persist even after several weeks. Tricyclics have lost some of their popularity to the newer SSRIs we describe earlier, because the SSRIs have fewer of these annoying side effects.

MAO inhibitors

MAO inhibitors are the oldest type of antidepressant medication. MAO inhibitors work by allowing critical neurotransmitters to remain available in the brain to effectively regulate mood. MAO inhibitors are used infrequently because they have serious side effects.

WARNING

Taking MAO inhibitors and consuming foods with tyramine can trigger a dangerous spike in blood pressure leading to stroke or death. Unfortunately, many foods, such as avocados, beer, cheese, salami, soy, wine, and tomatoes, contain tyramine.

Nevertheless, MAO inhibitors can be effective when other antidepressants haven't worked. If your doctor prescribes one of them for you, she probably has a good reason for doing so. However, watch what you eat, and ask your doctor for a complete list of foods to avoid, including those in the preceding list.

SAVING YOUR SEX LIFE?

Many medications for the treatment of anxiety, as well as depression, interfere with arousal and the ability to achieve an orgasm. The worst offenders in this group of medications are the SSRIs. Many folks taking these medications are so pleased with their reduced anxiety that they hesitate to complain to their doctors about this side effect. Others are just too embarrassed to bring it up.

You should know that this side effect is extremely common, and your doctor has no doubt heard many patients report this problem. So, go ahead and talk with your doctor — no need for embarrassment. Certain medications have a lower tendency to cause this side effect than others, so your doctor may recommend a switch. Alternatively, medications such as Viagra may be used to treat some of the sexual side effects directly. By talking to your doctor, you can explore the best options.

Benzodiazepines

Better known as tranquilizers, the benzodiazepines were first introduced in the 1960s. At first blush, these seemed like perfect medications for a host of anxiety problems. Unlike the antidepressants, they work rapidly, often reducing symptoms within 15 to 20 minutes. Not only that, they can be taken merely on an as-needed basis, when having to deal with an especially anxiety-arousing situation, such as confronting a phobia, giving a speech, or going to a job interview. The side effects tend to be less disturbing than those associated with antidepressants as well. And for many years after their introduction, they were seen as relatively safe with a low risk of overdose. They rapidly became the standard treatment for most of the anxiety disorders. They appear to work by reinforcing a substance in the brain that blocks the excitability of nerve cells. What could be better?

WARNING

Well, it turns out that the benzodiazepines do have some problems. Nothing's perfect, after all. Dependency or addiction is a particularly significant risk. As with many addictions, withdrawal from benzodiazepines can be difficult and even dangerous. Furthermore, if you stop taking them, your anxiety almost always returns. Rebound anxiety that's more severe than that experienced before taking the drug is possible upon withdrawal.

Benzodiazepines are also associated with increasing the risk of falling among the elderly. And falls among the elderly too often result in hip fractures. In addition, a recent report suggested that benzodiazepines may double the risk of getting into a motor vehicle accident.

That risk rapidly escalates when benzodiazepines are taken in combination with alcohol. In fact, benzodiazepines are particularly problematic for those who have a history of substance abuse. Those who are addicted to recreational drugs or alcohol readily become addicted to these medications and are at greater risk for taking dangerous combinations of drugs and alcohol that could result in an overdose.

TECHNICAL STUFF

Prescribing benzodiazepines to those who have suffered a recent trauma seems sensible and humane. And indeed, these medications have the potential to improve sleep and reduce both arousal and anxiety. However, some evidence has suggested that the early and prolonged administration of benzodiazepines after a trauma actually appeared to increase the rate of full-blown post-traumatic stress disorder (PTSD) later.

It seems logical to assume that combining benzodiazepines with some of the various changes in behavior, thinking, and acceptance that can reduce anxiety (see Chapters 5–9) would make for a useful combination that could yield a better outcome than using either approach by itself. Yet, studies have found that the risk of relapse is increased when these medications are combined with changes in thinking and behaving. In the long run, it appears that for most people, learning coping strategies to deal with their anxiety gets better results than merely seeking pharmacological solutions — especially with respect to the benzodiazepines.

Nevertheless, the benzodiazepines remain one of the most popular approaches to the treatment of anxiety disorders, especially among general practitioners who have no special training in psychiatry. In part, that may be due to the low side-effect profile of the drugs. And these medications can sometimes play an important role, especially for short-term, acute stress and anxiety, as well as for those for whom other medications haven't helped. We simply urge considerable caution with the use of these prescription drugs.

Miscellaneous tranquilizers

A few miscellaneous tranquilizers are chemically unrelated to the benzodiazepines and thus appear to work rather differently. These drugs may cause less addiction and are less likely to cause falls. However, they can sometimes lead to daytime fatigue, dizziness, and occasionally, anxiety.

TECHNICAL
STUFF

Although we don't list the myriad of specific drugs in this chapter, one has some unique benefits for certain types of anxiety and is worth mentioning. Buspar (buspirone) belongs to a class of chemical compounds referred to as *azaspirodecanediones* (which are actually far less intimidating than their name). It has been studied the most for the treatment of generalized anxiety disorder (GAD) but may have value for treating various other anxiety-related problems, such as social phobia and PTSD, among others. It may not be as useful for panic attacks as other medications. Buspar's primary benefits are that it's not likely to be addictive and causes less sedation than the benzodiazepines. Although extensive evidence is necessary to rule out addictive potential, the current belief is that Buspar's likelihood for producing dependence is quite low.

Beta blockers

Because anxiety can increase blood pressure, perhaps it's not surprising that a few medications for the treatment of hypertension also reduce anxiety. Chief among these are the so-called beta blockers that block the effects of norepinephrine (a chemical that gives the body extra energy for dealing with stress). Thus, they control many of the physical symptoms of anxiety, such as shaking, trembling, rapid heartbeat, and blushing. In the treatment of anxiety, their usefulness is primarily limited to specific phobias, such as social anxiety and performance anxiety. They're highly popular among professional musicians, who often use them to reduce their performance anxiety prior to an important concert or audition.

ATYPICAL ANTIPSYCHOTICS

Medications called *atypical antipsychotic medications* are not usually prescribed for anxiety disorders. They're atypical in the sense that, unlike earlier medications, they have a lower risk of certain serious side effects, and they can be used to treat a far broader range of problems than *psychosis*, a disturbance in the ability to perceive reality correctly. The atypical antipsychotics target a different neurotransmitter than the SSRIs and sometimes are used in combination with SSRIs. When used to treat anxiety-related problems, these medications are usually prescribed at far lower doses than when used for psychotic disorders.

These medications are primarily prescribed for people who have severe, hard-to-treat anxiety or who suffer from other mental disorders along with anxiety. They're generally not prescribed unless other forms of treatment have been unsuccessful. They have some especially distressing side effects. Possibly the most feared are known as extrapyramidal side effects (EPS), which can include a wide range of problems, such as

- Abnormal, uncontrollable, irregular muscle movements in the face, mouth, and, sometimes, other body parts
- An intense feeling of restlessness
- Muscle stiffness
- Prolonged spasms or muscle contractions
- Shuffling gait

These EPS effects appear to occur less often with the newer atypical antipsychotic medications as opposed to the older, traditional antipsychotic medications. However, because the risk exists, those with relatively milder anxiety problems would probably want to avoid them.

Warning: Another disturbing side effect with many of these atypical antipsychotics is a change in metabolism that increases the risk of weight gain and can eventually lead to diabetes. As with most of the medications for anxiety, these should generally be avoided when pregnant or breast-feeding. Consult your physician for the best alternatives.

Mood stabilizers

Mood stabilizers are usually prescribed for other conditions. However, when standard treatments haven't worked, doctors sometimes find them useful for treating their patients' anxiety. People who suffer mood swings like those with bipolar disorder often benefit from this particular class of drugs.

Medical marijuana

Marijuana for medical use is currently legal in many states, and recreational use has become legal in a growing number of states as well. There is substantial evidence that marijuana helps with chronic pain, decreases spasticity for people with multiple sclerosis (MS), and decreases chemotherapy induced nausea. There is limited scientific evidence that marijuana decreases anxiety and improves symptoms of PTSD. More research is needed.

Searching for Vitamins and Supplements

Dietary supplements include vitamins, amino acids, minerals, enzymes, metabolites, or botanicals that reputedly enhance your health and/or your body's functions. Such supplements appear in many different forms — capsules, powders, tablets, teas, liquids, and granules. You can buy supplements from the internet, your local drugstore, a grocery store, or a health food store. Claimed benefits of supplements include improved immune systems, enhanced sleep, stronger bones, revved-up sexual response, cancer cures, and overcoming anxiety.

WARNING

People seek supplements often because they assume that they're safer than prescription drugs. That's not necessarily true. Supplements are not considered drugs in the United States and therefore, are not subjected to the same level of scrutiny as most medications. Before a prescription drug can come to market, the manufacturer must conduct clinical studies to establish the safety, effectiveness, dosage, and possible harmful interactions with other medications. The U.S. Food and Drug Administration (FDA) doesn't require clinical trials to establish the safety of herbs. Instead, after a supplement makes it to market, the only way it will be removed is if enough consumers suffer serious side effects and complain to the right agencies, which can trigger an FDA investigation and possible decision to withdraw the herb from store shelves.

Other potential problems with supplements include

>> Adverse reactions that are not tracked by the FDA

>> Contaminants

>> Unknown, variable potency

>> Lack of controlled studies to verify their effectiveness

Another serious problem with supplements is that untrained salespeople often make recommendations for their use. Fortunately, healthcare professionals who are also interested and trained in the safe and effective use of supplements can help.

By contrast, salesclerks vary widely in the usefulness of their advice. Dolores's story isn't all that unusual.

A young, fit salesperson smiles at **Dolores** as she enters the health food store. Dolores tells him that she would like to find a natural remedy to help her calm down. She reports difficulty concentrating, poor sleep, and always feeling on edge. The young man nods and suggests a regimen of vitamins and supplements to build up her resistance to stress, improve her concentration, and ease her symptoms of anxiety.

Pulling bottles off the shelves, he tells her, "Some B vitamins to build you up; C to fight infections. Here are some amino acids — L-lysine and tyrosine — and a compound, 5-HTP. Melatonin for sleep. Oh yes, maybe some SAM-e to improve your mood. In addition, consider hops, passionflower, valerian, lemon balm, chamomile, and ashwagandha root. Now, take these at least an hour before you eat."

The bill comes to $314, and Dolores goes home feeling a bit overwhelmed. One day at work, after ingesting a dozen pills, she runs to the bathroom to throw up. A concerned friend asks her what's making her sick. Dolores tells her about all the supplements that she's taking. Her friend suggests that Dolores seek the advice of a nurse practitioner who specializes in wholistic medicine.

Dolores visits the nurse practitioner, who advises her to dump the majority of her purchases in favor of a single multiple vitamin and one herbal supplement. He also discusses psychotherapy, exercise routines, and self-help books. Within a few weeks, Dolores feels like a new person.

The example of Dolores may seem extreme. However, the supplement business is a highly profitable one. Well-intentioned salesclerks rarely have medical training.

Dolores was actually lucky compared to Hector, whose story appears next. Hector not only tries herbal supplements, but mixes them with a prescription drug and alcohol, resulting in a very dangerous scenario.

It's payday, and **Hector's** buddies invite him to hoist a few beers. "Sure," he says. "I can't stay too long, but I could use a beer; it's been a tough week." Munching on spicy bar mix, Hector finishes off his beer over the course of an hour. He stumbles a bit as he gets off the bar stool, and the bartender asks if he's okay. Hector reassures the bartender that he's sober. After all, he only had one beer.

Driving home, Hector drifts into the left lane for a moment but swerves back into line. Just then, he hears a car behind him honking. A few moments later, he sees police lights flashing. Puzzled, he pulls over. Hector fails a field sobriety test, but a breathalyzer test registers Hector's blood alcohol level at .02, well below the legal limit. What's going on?

Hector recently complained to his physician about feeling stressed at his job. His doctor prescribed a low dose of anti-anxiety medication and warned Hector not to take too much because it could be addictive if he wasn't careful. Hector found the medication useful, and it calmed him a bit, but the medication didn't quite do the trick. A friend recommended two herbs to try. Hector figured that would be a great, natural way to enhance the prescribed drug and that herbs certainly couldn't hurt him. To add up Hector's scorecard, he had combined two anxiety-alleviating herbs, a prescription drug, and alcohol — and was lucky that the police pulled him over. Hector could have ended up in a serious accident, harming himself or others.

WARNING

Don't forget that even low to moderate alcohol consumption combined with anti-anxiety agents can intensify sedative effects to the point of substantial impairment and even death. *Be careful!*

HUNTING FOR HELPFUL HERBS

People have used herbal remedies for thousands of years. Some of them work. In fact, a significant number of prescription medications are derived from herbs. You may want to try out an herb or two for your anxiety. We recommend that you read the literature about each herb carefully to make an informed choice before purchasing them from a reputable dealer. And always let your doctor know what herbs or supplements you're taking.

- **Saint John's Wort:** This plant has been used since ancient times for medicinal purposes. Research on St. John's Wort is insufficient to recommend this as a treatment for anxiety. Be careful: It can intensify the effects of sun and lead to sunburn. In addition, it may affect the liver and have the potential to cause dangerous interactions with other prescription drugs or alcohol.

- **Kava kava:** The islanders in the South Pacific have consumed kava kava for both pleasure and healing. They have typically used it to treat a host of ailments, including obesity, syphilis, and gonorrhea. The islanders have also used it for relaxation, insomnia, and anxiety reduction. Kava kava has been used extensively in Europe for anxiety, although usage varies from area to area. Studies suggest that it does have a positive effect on anxiety, although the effect is modest. However, a few countries have banned kava kava due to its reported potential for causing liver problems.

- **Valerian:** Valerian is an herb native to Europe and Asia. The word comes from the Latin term meaning *well-being*. Valerian has been suggested for digestive problems, insomnia, and anxiety. Like many herbs, it's used extensively in Europe but is gaining in popularity in the United States. However, research is limited on its efficacy for anxiety.

(continued)

(continued)

- **CBD (cannabidiol):** CBD is an active component found in cannabis plants. It is hugely popular throughout the United States. It can be found in various forms and concentrations in products such as candy, soft drinks, vape pens, and pills. The FDA has approved CBD for difficult-to-control epilepsy. CBD has been recommended as a help for anxiety, depression, inflammation, chronic pain, insomnia, Parkinson's disease, skin conditions, and more. These benefits are mostly reported by individuals and have not been well studied.

Many other herbal remedies for anxiety are promoted as safe, effective methods. But beware; most of these herbs haven't been subjected to scrutiny for effectiveness or safety. We suggest that you avoid these because so many other anxiety-reducing agents and strategies work without dangerous side effects. On the other hand, we don't think that you need to be overly alarmed about drinking a little herbal tea from time to time. Most of these brews contain relatively small amounts of the active ingredients and likely pose little threat.

Viva vitamins!

Chronic stress taxes the body. The results of several studies link mood disorders to vitamin deficiencies, and especially severe deficiencies may make your anxiety worse. Therefore, some experts recommend a good multivitamin supplement; however, that recommendation is increasingly uncommon. Research has simply failed to find much health benefit of taking vitamins regularly for the vast majority of people who take them. Can vitamins and minerals cure your anxiety? That's not likely.

WARNING

The vitamin and supplement business is a multi-billion-dollar enterprise. Half or more Americans take one or more vitamins or supplements regularly. For the most part, scientists believe consumers are wasting their money.

Sifting through the slew of supplements

If you search the internet and your local health food stores, you can probably find over a hundred supplements advertised as antidotes for anxiety. But do they work? Only a few that we know of. The following have at least garnered a smidge of evidence in support of their value as possible anxiety axes:

>> **Melatonin:** Reaching a peak around midnight, this hormone helps to regulate sleep rhythms in the body. In particular, it addresses the problem of falling asleep at the right time (known as sleep onset) as opposed to the problem of

awakening in the early morning and being unable to go back to sleep. Synthetic melatonin taken in the early evening, a few hours before bedtime, may alleviate this particular type of insomnia, a common problem among those who have excessive anxiety.

Side effects such as dizziness, irritability, fatigue, headache, and low-level depression are all possible, but the long-term side effects aren't really known at this time. Avoid driving or drinking alcohol when you take melatonin.

WARNING

If you have an autoimmune disease or if you're depressed, you should probably avoid melatonin.

>> **SAM-e:** Claimed to relieve the pain and stiffness of osteoarthritis and fibromyalgia, this amino acid occurs naturally in the body. It may also help treat depression and anxiety. However, research on this supplement remains limited. SAM-e appears to increase levels of serotonin and dopamine in the brain, which could theoretically alleviate anxiety.

Possible side effects such as gastrointestinal upset, nervousness, insomnia, headache, and agitation may result, but again, little is known about the possible long-term effects.

WARNING

Don't take SAM-e if you have bipolar disorder or severe depression. SAM-e may contribute to mania, which is a dangerous, euphoric state that often includes poor judgment and risky behaviors.

>> **5-HTP:** This popular supplement is a compound that increases the levels of serotonin in the brain. Serotonin plays a critical role in regulating mood and anxiety. Some evidence also exists that 5-HTP may increase the brain's natural pain relievers, *endorphins.* Unfortunately, only limited research has been conducted on this supplement. These studies suggest that 5-HTP may reduce anxiety and some report improved sleep.

WARNING

Don't take 5-HTP if you're also taking another antidepressant. Also, avoid it if you have tumors or cardiovascular disease.

>> **Omega-3 fatty acids:** Found in flax seed, avocados, soybeans, and fish, these acids have been shown to improve mood for those with depression. Evidence of their usefulness for anxiety is less robust, but there is some evidence that having enough omega 3 fatty acids in the body improves cardiovascular health. So, if you take Omega-3, make sure that it's purified to eliminate toxins like mercury.

Most herbal supplements are not widely supported by controlled research. Big pharmaceutical companies are not able to obtain patents for the use of supplements found in nature, therefore, they do not want to spend millions to do the necessary controlled research to substantiate claims of effectiveness. You should be skeptical of testimonials and proclamations promoting the latest "cure."

Stimulating the Brain

People with severe cases of anxiety often try many different treatments. Unfortunately, a very few cases neither resolve nor even improve with standard treatments such as psychotherapy or medication. For those people, advances in science and technology may offer hope for improvement or even a cure to their suffering.

Brain stimulation techniques from shock therapy to sophisticated, new neuro-stimulation techniques have offered some hope for people with chronic anxiety problems. You should be aware that the effectiveness of some of these new approaches has been reasonably confirmed, though further research is certainly called for. Although these techniques have been available and studied for decades, empirical support for their effectiveness remains modest. Psychotherapy clearly should be attempted prior to turning to brain stimulation.

Transcranial magnetic stimulation (TMS)

TMS involves inducing a magnetic field on the scalp by sending a small electrical current into a coil. This treatment does not require surgical implantation, so side effects are less dangerous than treatments that involve surgery.

TMS has mainly been used to treat depression. Various anxiety issues have also received some scrutiny with this approach. It's a popular treatment because it causes very few troubling side effects. Many more studies are needed to recommend TMS as a frontline treatment for people with anxiety. However, if you have had long-standing anxiety and tried unsuccessful treatments (including psycho-therapy), TMS may be something to consider.

Vagus nerve stimulation (VNS)

The vagus nerve sends information from the digestive system, the heart, and the lungs throughout the brain. Anxiety is usually experienced throughout these systems, with symptoms ranging from stomach upset to rapid breathing to feelings of fear to thinking that something bad may happen. VNS was developed as a treatment for people with epilepsy. A device is implanted in the chest that sends electric pulses to the vagus nerve.

This treatment has been found to help those with severe depression. Many of those who experienced relief from either epileptic seizures or depression also noted decreases in anxiety. Therefore, a few studies have been conducted using VNS with treatment-resistant cases of anxiety. Results are minimally hopeful, but considerably more research is needed. For now, VNS remains an alternative primarily for those who have had multiple treatment failures for severe anxiety.

WARNING

Although serious side effects are rare, VNS can cause pain at the site of the incision, voice hoarseness, sore throat, and facial muscle weakness.

3 Letting Go of the Battle

IN THIS PART . . .

Embrace your family and friends.

Dive into delegation.

Extend yourself with exercise.

Tuck yourself in for a good night's sleep.

Develop a healthy diet.

Chapter **11**

Looking at Lifestyle

D o you lead a busy life with too much to do and too little time? Do you grab dinner from the nearest drive-through for you and the kids on the way home from soccer practice? Do you lie awake at night thinking about everything you have to do? Your frantic lifestyle probably leads to poor sleep, not enough exercise, and poor diet. You know you should be taking better care of yourself, which makes you feel stressed and anxious, compounding the problem.

In this chapter, we describe three sound strategies for calming down your life: staying connected with others, delegating, and saying "no." We also help you find the motivation for bringing exercise into your life. We show you how to get the best rest possible and what to do in the hours before bed that can help your sleep. Finally, we take a look at some tips for improving eating habits to quell anxious feelings.

Friends and Family — Can't Live with 'em, Can't Live without 'em

Some days, the people in your life provide all the love and support you could ever want. They offer to do things for you, listen to your woes, and comfort you when things go wrong. Other days, those same people make you wish you could move to a deserted island for a couple of weeks. They make unreasonable demands and lean on you excessively — complaining about problems of their own making, leaving you feeling stressed and worn out. The following three sections discuss the pros and cons of people in your life and offer suggestions on how to get the most out of your relationships.

Staying connected to others

In spite of the potential of family and friends to cause stress and aggravation, numerous studies have demonstrated that good, close relationships greatly enhance people's sense of well-being. Staying connected with people pays off in terms of substantially improved mental and physical health. Connections even appear to provide some protection against mental declines that often accompany old age.

TIP

So, we highly recommend that you focus on friendship, community, and family bonds—even when they're imperfect. Here are a few ideas for doing so:

>> Make sure you make time for face-to-face contact with your friends — don't just connect with them on social media.

>> Have family meals together whenever possible — it doesn't have to be any fancier than ordering pizza.

>> Volunteer at a nearby Humane Society, hospital, or school.

>> Call a friend you haven't talked with in a while.

>> Take walks in your neighborhood and introduce yourself to people you encounter.

>> Offer to help your family members with a garage sale or some other project.

You get the idea. Staying connected doesn't have to take lots of time or cost money, but it does take effort. That effort pays off not only for you but also for your friends, family, and community.

TIP

If your community is in the middle of a pandemic and there are restrictions on getting together, there are modifications that you can make to the preceding activities. Wear a mask, stay socially distant, and wash your hands frequently. For example, meet in a park, take your own food and drink, stay socially distant, and have a picnic.

REMEMBER

One connection involves you and at least one other person. So, when you reach out to someone else, you may be doing them just as much good as you're doing yourself.

What's that? You say you don't have time to connect with friends and family members? We've got solutions for that problem in the next two sections.

Delegating for extra time

Many people with anxiety feel they must always take responsibility for their job, the care of their family, and their home. Unless they have a hand in everything, they worry that things may not get done. And if someone else takes over a task, they fear that the result will fall short of their standards.

However, if life has become overwhelming and too stressed, learning to delegate may be your only choice. Pushing yourself too hard can put you at risk for illness, bad moods, and increased anxiety. And delegating a few things usually works out much better than you think it will.

TIP

Here are a few possibilities for your delegating list:

>> Take the risk of asking your partner to do housework or some other task that he or she doesn't normally do.

>> Hire a cleaning service to come in twice a year for spring and fall cleanup. It's a real treat. Do it more often if you can afford it.

>> Spend a Sunday afternoon as a family preparing large quantities of a few meals that can be frozen and consumed over the next week and much later.

>> Enlist the family to spend one hour a week in a frantic, joint cleaning effort. Listen to loud music while you clean.

>> Hire a monthly lawn service.

>> Have each member of the family plan and cook a meal every week.

We realize a few of these ideas cost money. Not always as much as you may think, but still, they do cost something. Partly, it's a matter of how high money stacks up on your priority list. Balance money against time for the things that you value.

Nevertheless, not all families can consider such options. You may notice that not all these options entail financial burden. Get creative. Ask your friends, co-workers, and family for ideas on how to delegate. It could change your life.

TIP

Come up with two tasks that you can delegate to someone else. They don't need to cost money — just relieve one or more of your burdens in a way that saves you time.

Just saying "no"

We have one more idea. Say "no." If you're anxious, you may have trouble standing up for your rights. Anxiety often prevents people from expressing their feelings and needs. When that happens, resentment joins anxiety and leads to frustration and anger. Furthermore, if you can't say "no," other people can purposefully or inadvertently take advantage of you. You no longer own your time and your life.

First, notice the situations in which you find yourself agreeing when you don't really want to. Does it happen mostly at work, with family, with friends, or with strangers? When people ask you to do something, try the following:

» **Validate the person's request or desire.** For example, if someone asks you if you'd mind dropping off something at the post office on your way home from work, say, "I understand that it would be more convenient for you if I dropped that off." This will give you more time to consider whether you really want to do it.

» **After you make up your mind to say "no," look the person who's making the request in the eye.** You don't need to rush your response.

» **Give a brief explanation, especially if it's a friend or family member.** However, remember that you really don't owe anyone an explanation for turning down their request; it's merely polite. You can say that you'd like to help out, but it just isn't possible, or you can simply state that you really would rather not.

» **Be clear that you can't or won't do what you've been asked.** It's a fundamental human right to say "no."

TIP

When you say "no" to bosses or family members, they may be temporarily unhappy with you. If you find yourself overreacting to their displeasure, it may be due to an anxious assumption. See Chapter 7 for more information about anxious assumptions.

Ready . . . Exorcise!

Please excuse our pun: We're not advising that you attempt to exorcise demons or perform hocus-pocus, but like a good housecleaning, exercise can clear out the cobwebs and cast out the cloudy thinking and inertia that may accompany anxiety.

Exercise reduces anxiety. The harder and longer that you go at it — whether you're swimming, jogging, walking, working in the yard or on your home, playing racquetball or tennis, or even walking up the stairs — the less anxious you'll be. Exercise instills a newfound sense of confidence while blowing away anxiety's cloud. With enough exercise, you'll feel your attitude changing from negative to positive.

Adults need about 150 minutes a week of moderate exercise to achieve benefits. That's less than 30 minutes a day. Moderate means brisk walking, slow jogging, swimming, or doing vigorous household chores. You can break those down into 10- or 15-minute stints. It doesn't matter. The point is to get up and move — often.

Some people with anxiety get a little driven and compulsive. Don't take our advice on exercise and go overboard! Yes, the more, the better, but only to a point. If your exercise starts taking time from other important activities, you may be overdoing it.

Exercise reduces anxiety in several ways:

>> It helps to rid your body of the excess adrenaline that increases anxiety and arousal.

>> It increases your body's production of *endorphins* — substances that reduce pain and create a mild, natural sense of well-being.

>> It helps to release muscle tension and frustrations.

Of course, everyone has felt that they should exercise more. Most people realize that exercise has some sort of health benefits, but not everyone knows how extensive these benefits can be. Researchers have found that exercise decreases anxiety, bad cholesterol, blood pressure, depression, and chronic pain. It also decreases risks of various diseases, such as heart disease and some cancers. Finally, exercise strengthens bones and improves your immune system, muscle and joint function, balance, flexibility, mental sharpness, memory, and sense of well-being.

Wow! With such extensive positive effects on anxiety, health, and well-being, why isn't everyone exercising? Millions of people do. Unfortunately, millions do not. The reasons are both simple and complex. For the most part, people hit a brick wall when it comes to finding the motivation to exercise and especially to sustain it. They complain about not having the time and being too embarrassed, too old, too fat, and too tired to exercise.

But if our list of benefits appeals to you, the next section, "Don't wait for willpower — Just do it!" may help you muster the motivation. And then, because we know what you're going to think next — "I don't have time to exercise!" — we provide a list of excuse-busting ways to fit your workout into your schedule.

Before beginning an exercise program, you should check with your doctor. This is especially true if you're over 40, overweight, or have any known health problems. Your doctor can tell you about any cautions, limitations, or restrictions that you should consider. Also, if, after brief exercise, you experience chest pain, extreme shortness of breath, nausea, or dizziness, consult your physician immediately.

Don't wait for willpower — Just do it!

Have you ever thought that you just don't have the willpower to undertake an exercise program? You may be surprised to discover that we don't believe in willpower. That's right. *Willpower* is merely a word, an idea; it's not real.

Your brain doesn't have a special structure that contains so-called willpower. It's not something that you have a set quantity of and that you can't do anything about. The reason people believe that they don't have willpower is merely because they don't do what they think they should.

Nevertheless, willpower is a powerful concept or idea that almost everyone believes in. And if you change its meaning to refer to willingness to exert effort on something, maybe it makes a certain amount of sense. But reasons other than willpower actually account for that lack of effort: namely, distorted thinking and a failure to include sufficient rewards. Therefore, dealing with distorted thoughts and designing rewards works better than waiting for willpower.

Distorted thinking

Your mind may tell you things like, "I just don't have the time," "I'm too tired," "It isn't worth the effort," or "I'll look stupid compared to the other people who are in better shape than me."

If you have thoughts like these, first realize that they're just thoughts. Just because you think something, doesn't make it true. Challenge those thoughts with something more encouraging. See Chapter 6 for lots more information about how to challenge your distorted thinking. You don't want distorted thoughts to run your life.

If you're waiting for motivation to come knocking at your door, you could be in for a long wait. Not many people wake up with a burst of new enthusiasm for starting an exercise program. Like the Nike slogan says, "Just do it." That's because motivation frequently *follows* action; if you think otherwise, you're putting the cart before the horse.

Lack of reward

Another problem that accounts for lack of motivation comes about when you fail to set up a plan for rewarding new efforts. You may believe that exercise will cost you something in terms of leisure time, rest, or more profitable work. In some ways, this is true. That's why you need to set up a plan for reinforcing your efforts.

Psychologists have known for decades that people usually do more of what they find rewarding and less of what they find unpleasant whenever they can. That fact may sound like a no-brainer to you. Nevertheless, ignoring the importance of rewards is easy when trying to get started on an exercise program.

Set up your own personal reward system for exercising. For example, give yourself ten points for each time that you exercise for 15 minutes, or more. After you accumulate 100 points, indulge yourself with a treat — buying a new outfit, going out for dinner at a nice restaurant, planning a special weekend, or setting aside a whole day to spend on your favorite hobby. Over time, as exercise becomes a little more pleasant (which it will!), up the ante — require 200 points before you treat yourself.

Eventually, you'll find that exercise becomes rewarding in its own right, and you won't need to reward yourself as a means of instilling the necessary motivation. As the pain of an out-of-shape body lessens and endurance increases, you'll discover other rewards from exercise as well:

>> It can be a great time to think about solutions to problems.

>> You can plan out the day or week while you exercise.

>> Some people report increased creative thoughts during exercise.

>> You'll get a great feeling from the sense of accomplishment.

>> Once you get into better shape, you'll feel better physically and emotionally.

Because exercise often doesn't feel good in the beginning, setting up a self-reward system sometimes helps a great deal; later, other rewards will kick in.

Working in your workout

Today, people work longer hours than ever before, so it's tempting to think that the day doesn't hold enough time for exercise. However, it's all a matter of priorities; you won't find the time unless you plan for it.

That's right; you have to scrutinize your schedule seriously, and work exercise into your life. Perhaps your job offers flex time, whereby you can choose to come in an hour later and stay later two or three times a week to have time to exercise in the morning, or perhaps you can exercise twice on the weekends and find just one time after work during the week. And, it isn't all that difficult to add a little to your regular exercise periods. For example:

>> **Park at a distance:** Park your car about a 20-minute brisk walk away from your place of work once or twice a week.

>> **Take the stairs:** If you often take the elevator up five or six floors to work, try a brisk walk up the stairs several times a day instead.

HOW ABOUT EXERCISE AND PANIC?

Some people fear that exercise could set off panic attacks. In part, that's because exercise produces a few bodily symptoms, such as increased heart rate, that are similar to the symptoms of panic attacks, and those with a panic disorder sometimes respond to such symptoms with panic. However, if you go at exercise gradually, it can serve as a graded exposure task, as we discuss in Chapter 9. In other words, it can be an effective treatment approach for panic.

Although the actual risk is somewhat controversial, exercise can cause a buildup of lactic acid, which does seem to trigger panic attacks in a few people. However, over the long run, exercise also improves your body's ability to rid itself of lactic acid. Therefore, again, we recommend that if you fear having panic attacks as a result of exercise, simply go slowly. If you find it absolutely intolerable, stop exercising for a while or use other strategies in this book for reducing your panic attack frequency before going back to exercise.

>> **Exercise during your breaks:** If you get a couple of 10- or 15-minute breaks at work, try going for a brisk walk rather than standing around the water cooler. Two or three 10-minute periods of exercise do you the same amount of good as that one 20- or 30-minute period does.

>> **Consider high intensity interval training (HIIT).** You can find seven-minute workouts on the internet that can help you burn calories, increase metabolism, and improve cardiovascular health.

TIP

A variety of studies support the value of exercise in helping most people manage their anxiety. When you're exercising vigorously, it's difficult to be immersed in ruminations about what's bothering you. Like we've said, just do it.

The ABCs of Getting Your Zs

People generally need about eight hours of sleep per night. Seniors may need a little less sleep, and there are individual exceptions. The real gauge as to whether you're getting enough sleep is how you feel during the daytime, not the exact number of hours you get. In any case, anxiety frequently disrupts sleep, and a lack of sleep can increase your anxiety.

Many people have trouble falling asleep at night. As if falling asleep isn't hard enough, many people wake up before they want to, driven into high alert as anxious thoughts race through their consciousness.

There are some realistic reasons that not getting enough sleep causes anxiety. People who have chronic sleep deprivation tend to be pessimistic, have impaired memory, have emotional outbursts, gain weight, and have suppressed immune systems.

WARNING

The tendency toward an early-morning awakening with an inability to get back to sleep can be a sign of depression as well as anxiety. If your appetite changes, your energy decreases, your mood swings into low gear, your ability to concentrate diminishes, and you've lost interest in activities that you once found pleasurable, you may be clinically depressed. You should check with a mental health practitioner or a physician to find out.

More goes into sleeping than just lying down and shutting your eyes. Factors that affect your sleep include the activities you do before you go to bed, your sleeping environment, and knowing what to do when sleep is elusive. We address these topics in the following sections.

Creating a sleep haven

Your sleep environment matters. Of course, some rare birds can sleep almost anywhere — on the couch, in a chair, on the floor, in the car, or even at their desk at work. On the other hand, most folks require the comfort of a bed and the right conditions. Sleep experts report that for a restful sleep, you should sleep in a room that's

TIP

>> **Dark:** You have a clock in your brain that tells you when it's time to sleep. Darkness helps set the clock by causing the brain to release melatonin, a hormone that helps to induce sleep. Consider putting up curtains that block out most of the sun if you find yourself awakened by the early morning light, or you need to sleep during the day. Some people wear masks to keep light out.

>> **Cool:** People sleep better in a cool room. If you feel cold, adding blankets is usually preferable to turning up the thermostat.

>> **Quiet:** If you live near a busy street or have loud neighbors, consider getting a fan or use a white noise app on your phone to block out nuisance noises. The worst kind of noise is intermittent and unpredictable. If the noise is disturbing, the various kinds of sporadic noise that can be blocked out by a simple floor fan may amaze you.

>> **Complete with a comfortable bed:** Mattresses matter. Get pillows that you like. If you sleep with someone else or a dog, make sure that everyone has enough room.

In other words, make your bedroom a retreat that looks inviting and cozy. Spoil yourself with high-thread-count sheets and pillowcases. You may want to try aromatherapy. No one knows for sure whether it works, but many people claim that the fragrance of lavender helps them sleep.

Turn off the notifications on your phone, and please don't be tempted to look at the screen for more than a moment after you're in bed. The light from the phone can disturb your circadian rhythm.

Following a few relaxing routines

Sleep revitalizes your physical and mental resources. Studies show that sleep deprivation causes people to drive as if they were under the influence of drugs or alcohol. Physicians without sufficient sleep make more errors. Sleep deprivation makes you irritable, crabby, anxious, and despondent.

Thus, you need to schedule a reasonable amount of time for sleep — at least seven or eight hours. Don't burn the candle at both ends. We don't care how much work you have on your plate; depriving yourself of sleep only makes you less productive and less pleasant to be around.

So first and foremost, allow sufficient time for sleep. But that's not enough if you have trouble with sleep, so we suggest that you look at the ideas in the subsections that follow to improve the quality of your sleep.

Whenever possible, go to bed at close to the same time every night. Many people like to stay up late on weekends, and that's fine if you're not having sleep problems, but if you are, we recommend sticking to the same schedule you follow on weeknights. You need a regular routine to prepare your mind for bed.

Associating sleep with your bed

One of the most important principles of sleep is to teach your brain to associate sleep with your bed. That means that when you get into bed, don't bring work along with you. Some people find that reading before bed relaxes them, and others like to watch a little TV before bed. That's fine if these activities work for you, but generally, avoid doing them in bed.

If you go to bed and lie there for more than 20 or 30 minutes unable to fall asleep, get up. Again, the point is to train your brain to link your bed to sleep. You can train your brain to dislike getting up by taking on some unpleasant (though fairly passive, even boring) chore while you're awake. Or some people find that it works for them to get up and just get a sip of milk or water. The point is to get up so you can associate your bed with sleep rather than not sleeping. If you do this a number of times, your brain will find it easier to start feeling drowsy when you're in bed.

Winding down before hitting the hay

TIP

Some people find that taking a warm bath with fragrant oils or bath salts about an hour before hitting the hay is soothing. You may discover that soaking in a scented bath in a dimly lit bathroom while listening to relaxing music before going to bed is just the right ticket to solid slumber. Others may find reading, meditating, or straightening up the kitchen relaxing. Studies show that the induction of a relaxed state can improve sleep.

WARNING

You need to wind down with passive activities before you turn in for the night. Therefore, don't do heavy exercise within a few hours of going to sleep. Almost any stimulating activity can interfere with sleep, even mental exertion. For example, many people find that watching the news, engaging in most types of work, reading an emotionally intense book, or watching a highly engaging movie or television series disturbs their ability to fall asleep.

Watching what you eat and drink

Obviously, you don't want to load up on caffeinated drinks within a couple of hours before going to bed. Don't forget that many sources other than coffee — colas, certain teas, chocolate, and certain pain relievers — contain caffeine. Of course, some people seem rather impervious to the effects of caffeine while others are better off not consuming any after lunch. Even if you haven't been bothered by caffeine in the past, you can develop sensitivity to it as you age. Consider caffeine's effects on you if you're having trouble sleeping.

Nicotine also revs up the body. Try to avoid smoking just prior to bed. Obviously, it's preferable to quit smoking entirely, but if you haven't been able to stop yet, at least watch how much you smoke before bedtime. If you need help with an engrained smoking habit, consider getting a copy of Quitting Smoking & Vaping For Dummies by yours truly (Wiley).

WARNING

Alcohol relaxes the body and should be a great way of aiding sleep, but it isn't. That's because alcohol disrupts your sleep cycles. You don't get as much of the important REM sleep, and you may find yourself waking up early in the morning. However, some people find that drinking a glass of wine in the evening is relaxing. That's fine, but watch the amount.

Heavy meals prior to bed aren't such a great idea either; many people find that eating too much before bed causes mild discomfort. In addition, you may want to avoid highly spiced and/or fatty foods prior to bed. However, going to bed hungry is also a bad idea; the key is balance.

TIP

So, what should you eat or drink before bed? Herbal teas, such as chamomile or valerian, have many advocates. We don't have much data on how well they work, but herbal teas are unlikely to interfere with sleep, and they're pleasant to drink. Some evidence supports eating a small carbohydrate snack before bedtime to help induce sleep.

Mellowing with medication

Some people try treating their sleep problems with over-the-counter medications, many of which contain antihistamines that do help, but they can lead to drowsiness the next day. Occasional use of these medications is relatively safe for most. Herbal formulas, such as melatonin or valerian, may also help.

If your sleep problems are chronic, you should consult your doctor. A medication that you're already taking could be interfering with your sleep. Your doctor may prescribe medication to help induce sleep. Many sleep medications become less effective over time, and some carry the risk of addiction. These potentially addictive medications are only used for a short period of time. On the other hand, a few sleep medications work as sleep aids for a longer time without leading to addiction. Talk about your sleep problem with your doctor for more information and help.

Taking action when sleep just won't come

If you've been practicing the suggestions in the previous sections and still haven't resolved your sleep problems, we have a few more suggestions. Becky's story illustrates some of the problematic thoughts people have that keep them awake. Then we tell you what to do about them.

> As the clock chimes the hour, **Becky** sighs, realizing that it's 2 a.m., and she has yet to fall asleep. She turns over and tries to be still so that she doesn't wake her husband. She thinks, "With everything I have to do tomorrow, if I don't sleep, I'll be a wreck. I hate not sleeping." She gets out of bed, goes into the bathroom, finds the bottle of melatonin, and pops three into her mouth. She's been taking them routinely for months, and they just don't seem to have the same effect that they did before.
>
> She goes back to bed, tries to settle down, and worries about the bags under her eyes and what people will think. Her itchy, dry skin starts to crawl. She can't stand the feeling of lying in bed for an eternity without sleeping.

In Becky's mind, her lack of sleep turns into a catastrophe, and her pondering actually makes it far more difficult for her to fall asleep.

TIP

When you can't sleep, try to make the problem seem less catastrophic by

>> **Reminding yourself that every single time that you failed to sleep in the past, somehow you got through the next day in spite of your lack of sleep the night before.** It may not have been wonderful, but you did it.

>> **Realizing that occasional sleep loss happens to everyone.** Excessive worry can only aggravate the problem.

>> **Getting up and distracting yourself with something else.** This stops your mind from magnifying the problem and can also prevent you from associating your bed with not sleeping.

>> **Concentrating solely on your breathing.** Spend some time counting your breaths — it works better than counting sheep.

WARNING

Many people try taking daytime naps when they consistently fail to sleep at night. It sounds like a great solution, but unfortunately, it only compounds the problem. Frequent or prolonged naps disrupt your body's natural clock. If you must nap, make it a short power nap — no longer than 20 minutes.

Of course, a few unusual folks find that they can nap for just three or four minutes whenever they want during the day; they wake up refreshed and sleep well at night. If that's you, go ahead and nap. Most people simply can't do that.

TIP

If nothing seems to work for you, consider looking for a professional who has skills in using cognitive behavior therapy for insomnia. Getting enough sleep is important for everyone, especially those who are trying to work on their anxiety. You need the energy and stamina that sleep provides.

Designing Calm Diets

Uncomfortable emotions cause some people to eat too much, others to seek so-called comfort food (full of fat and sugar), and still others to lose their appetites. Unfortunately, emotional eating only works for the very short run — perhaps a few minutes to an hour or so. In the long run, bad dieting habits increase distress either from weight gain or the negative impact on your body due to spikes in blood sugar levels or irregularity. So, we recommend that you follow a few simple, well-known principles of good eating to stabilize both your body and mind.

Enjoying small, frequent portions

Portion sizes have expanded almost as dramatically as people's waistlines over the past century. Your great grandmother's china appears doll-sized by today's standards. In fact, some antique dealers report having trouble convincing customers that grandma's dinner plates really are dinner plates and not for bread or salad.

By and large, most people simply eat too much at one time today. Here are a few ways to control portions:

TIP

» **Use smaller plates:** This creates an optical illusion, and you think you're eating more food than you really are.

» **Eat slowly:** This gives your stomach time to tell your brain that you're full and should stop eating.

» **Fill your plate once, and put away the leftovers before you start eating:** This reduces the temptation to go back for seconds.

» **When you're at a restaurant, split a meal with a friend or box up half of it before you start eating:** Restaurant portions are typically twice the size they should be for one meal. Eating only half of the meal provides the right amount of calories.

In other words, plan out what you want to eat, and slow down your eating. Prepare several small, healthy snacks for dealing with cravings during the day.

Following nutritional common sense

For many people, the feeling of anxiety is similar to hunger. When stressed, a bowl of ice cream or some French fries with lots of ketchup sounds yummy, and those foods can momentarily boost moods. That's because they contain loads of simple carbohydrates. The body turns those carbs into sugar and burns it up like rocket fuel — really fast. That fast burn then leads to a rapid drop in blood sugar levels, often leading to a plunging mood, irritability, and a return of sugar cravings.

Replacing those simple carbohydrates with food containing complex carbs and fiber maintains stable blood sugar levels and a stable mood. Complex carbs are found in unprocessed foods, fruits, vegetables, whole grains, and legumes.

TIP

Good diets are fairly easy to find on the web. The Mediterranean Diet is considered one of the healthiest diets. Common sense tells you what to do — eat a variety of whole foods, and stay away from junk. The take-home message is to not make food an extra source of stress in your life.

Chapter **12**

Meditating as Part of a Healthy Lifestyle

Meditation is a difficult concept to define. That's because there are so many varieties of meditation, and procedures vary even within a given type. Meditation *usually* involves focused attention, a quiet location without distractions, a still position, and an open mind. Just a few problems: Some meditation occurs while a person is walking, people may meditate in a noisy airport, sometimes attention meanders, and thoughts may readily intrude. Skepticism may even show up. So, meditation is different for different people. There is no specific, universally agreed upon definition or set of strategies for meditation.

In spite of all these differences, the field of mental health has witnessed a substantial uptick in professional and scientific interest in meditation. Research findings have supported a range of significant benefits from meditation. In this chapter, we give you a brief look at what meditation does and what it helps with. We introduce you to some of the major types of meditation. Finally, we give you tips on how to master techniques and some cautions about what to avoid.

TECHNICAL STUFF

As we note in this chapter, meditation has been determined to be effective for a variety of health and well-being purposes. However, a limitation of this research has been the difficulty in comparing different meditation strategies. That's because some techniques involve chanting, some counting, some are 10 minutes in length, others are 30 minutes, or longer. So, it's like comparing apples and

oranges. Nevertheless, enough research has been conducted to support the mental and physical health benefits of a variety of meditation strategies.

Meditation Basics

Our first encounter with formal meditation training began in the 1990s. The lessons were given in an old adobe house along an acequia (irrigation ditch) in a small New Mexico town. The instructor was a martial arts and yogi master whose calm, assured manner provided much-needed confidence for the novice class. We sat on small flat cushions on polished wood floors, in front of a pleasant wood fire.

During the first session, we learned how to sit — cross-legged with hands perched lightly on the knees. After a few minutes, body parts started to cramp. The master told us to expect discomfort at first, but breathe through it. We weren't sure how to do that but stayed silent. We learned to take cleansing breaths and how to focus our attention on breathing. After a few sessions, we started using mantras.

Both of us still recall the warm room with our master's booming, deep, vibrating voice intoning, "ohm, ahh, umm." While we sat attempting to imitate, we also experienced a crescendo of intrusive thoughts. They were mostly along these lines

>> My foot is cramping.

>> This is uncomfortable.

>> My nose itches.

>> I shouldn't be having all these thoughts,

>> So, with eight people each paying $50, he's sure making a lot of money teaching this class.

>> I wonder what time it is.

>> Do we really need to do this 45 minutes every day?

>> I have to pick up the laundry and take the dog to the vet before it closes.

>> I'm not getting better at this.

>> What am I doing wrong?

>> Is this really worth $50 an hour?

>> How much longer until we finish today? I don't want to look at my watch.

The class met twice a week for six weeks. We just couldn't see re-enrolling. Meditation dropouts. How sad.

Since we were professional, clinical psychologists, we didn't talk too much about our experience with meditation. In part, that's because meditation was only starting to catch on among mental health professionals as a possible mainstream treatment for problems like anxiety and chronic pain. So, our dropout status wasn't a big concern. But nothing to brag about either.

However, times have changed in the intervening years since our initial foray into meditation. Today, meditation is a common tool used in self-help and to supplement psychotherapy, and is frequently suggested as part of a healthy lifestyle.

By the way, since the 1990s we've reconnected with meditation practice through workshops, training, and our own personal practice. We've learned much, and now meditation is a regular part of our lives.

What's So Good About Meditating?

Meditation has been around for centuries. With that kind of staying power, you almost have to figure there's something good about it. But we're skeptical scientists, so we like it when research studies concur with popular opinion. Science indeed backs up the value of meditation. Research has shown you are likely to benefit in some of the following ways if you incorporate meditation into your lifestyle:

>> **Anxiety:** Reviews of numerous studies have demonstrated that you can expect moderate improvement in symptoms from regular meditation.

>> **Stress:** Meditation has been shown to improve the ability to cope.

>> **Depression:** Some evidence suggests that meditation helps decrease levels of depression and is particularly helpful in preventing relapse.

>> **Physical health:** Studies have generally shown that meditation decreases blood pressure, decreases inflammatory responses, improves the ability to cope with chronic pain, and reduces the severity of gastrointestinal symptoms.

>> **Memory:** New research has shown early promise in facilitating memory.

>> **Thinking:** Meditation appears to improve attention and decrease a tendency to dwell and ruminate on disturbing thoughts.

>> **Insomnia:** Meditation improves sleep (including onset and nighttime awakening).

With such a list of likely benefits, we suggest you give it a trial run. You don't have to pay a guru to begin a meditation practice.

Meditation Methods

Everyone who meditates brings something of themselves into their practice. And meditation itself comes in a variety of types and forms. Before we describe a few of those types, we have a few general suggestions that we've found helpful:

>> Find a relatively quiet place but realize that sounds very well may intrude, and that's alright. Obviously, it's a good idea to turn off your devices.

>> Wear comfortable clothes that allow unrestricted breathing and movement.

>> Find a comfortable position and rest your hands on your lap or knees.

>> Realize that any number of thoughts may float through. Accept them as mere thoughts moving through your mind.

>> Let go of your desire to judge how well you're doing. Just practicing meditation is success enough.

>> Focus on present moment experiencing rather than evaluating the past or future.

>> If you have discomfort, you may practice accepting it or simply readjust your position, scratch your nose, or do whatever you want to do.

>> Realize there are no absolute rights or wrongs about most forms of meditation.

Please note that your beginning meditation efforts may be easier if you find a person or recording that guides your practice. Some people prefer guided meditation, whereas others like to wing it on their own.

TIP

We've found that many novices are quite surprised to discover that meditation can be so permissive. They envisioned rigid rules and structure that must be adhered to precisely.

Breathing meditation

Breathing meditation is a form of meditation in which there is a focus on the breath. A focus on the breath is also a part of many other major forms of meditation. We treat it separately here so you can experience what it feels like. Here's a sample of how you go about breathing meditation:

1. **Take several long, deep breaths.**

2. **Gently close your eyes.**

   Be aware of your experience of breathing. Feel the air as it enters your nose or mouth. Notice the movement of your chest and belly. Notice the air as you exhale.

3. **Attend to your breathing.**

   If you have thoughts, let them go as if they were leaves floating down a stream or clouds moving across the sky.

4. **Slowly breathe in and breathe out.**

   If you're having discomfort, you can bring your awareness to it without changing it. If you want to shift your position, that's okay, too.

5. **Breathe in and out in your own rhythm.**

   Notice your breath. No need to change anything. Accept thoughts, sounds, sensations, and other distractions for what they are.

6. **Return to your breathing — in and out.**

   No need to judge anything. Just feel and experience your breath.

You can practice breathing meditation for five or ten minutes, or even an hour or longer. Many people count their breaths as a way to aid focus. When you notice your thoughts drifting, return to the breath when you can.

Body scan meditation

Body scan meditation has often been used effectively for people who have chronic pain. You can practice body scan either sitting or lying down. The following is an example of body scan procedures:

1. **Take a few slow, deep breaths, and gently close your eyes.**

2. **Notice your body. Feel the weight of your body on the floor or the seat of your chair.**

3. **Take a few more deep breaths.**

   Bring in more oxygen to enliven the body. As you exhale, relax more deeply.

4. **Move your awareness to your feet.**

   Notice the weight, the pressure, the temperature. Are they hot or cold?

5. **Now move your awareness slowly up your legs to your knees.**

   Relax your knees. If you feel pain or discomfort, breathe, and accept those sensations. You may alter your position if that feels right to you.

6. **Move your attention through your thighs and up to your stomach.**

   Let your stomach muscles soften and return focus to your breath.

7. **Notice your back pressing against the floor or the chair. Relax your shoulders.**

8. **Feel your hands. Allow your hands and arms to relax.**

9. **Move your awareness to your neck and head.**

   Relax your neck, soften your eyes, relax your forehead.

10. **Scan your entire body, and accept whatever sensations you feel.**

    Breathe in and out. Breathe in and out. When you are ready, slowly open your eyes.

TIP

This body scan sample is relatively brief. Most are considerably longer but retain the essence of what we present here. You can get scripts for body scan meditation by searching for "body scan script" on the internet.

Tasting meditation

How many times have you eaten a meal and barely tasted it? Of course, if it tastes like microwaved cardboard, perhaps that's a good thing. However, most of the foods that we eat taste pretty good. What a shame to miss out on the full experience.

TIP

Choose a time to practice an eating meditation. Be sure it's not a ten-minute lunch. But it doesn't require hours, either. Worrisome thoughts may sometimes distract you. That's fine and normal. However, try merely noticing them. Rather than judge those thoughts or yourself, return your focus to your eating when you can. Follow these steps:

1. **Slow down, and focus before taking a bite.**

2. **Look at your food.**

   Notice how it's displayed on your plate or bowl. Observe the food's colors, textures, and shapes.

3. **Take time to smell the aroma.**

   Put a small portion on your fork or spoon. Before you take a bite, hold it briefly under your nose.

4. **Briefly put the food on your lips and then on the tip of your tongue.**

5. **Put the food in your mouth, but don't bite down for a moment or two.**

6. **Chew very slowly.**

   Notice how the taste and texture change with each bite, and how the food tastes on different parts of your tongue.

7. **Swallow the bite, and notice how it feels sliding down your throat.**

8. **Follow this procedure throughout your meal.**

9. **Stay seated at the table with your meal for at least 20 minutes.**

   If you finish eating before the 20 minutes are up, continue sitting until the full 20 minutes have elapsed, and notice your surroundings and the sensations in your body.

Consider making eating meditation a regular part of your life. You'll feel calmer, enjoy your food more, and possibly even lose a little weight. Many weight-loss programs suggest slowing down your eating. However, this approach does more — it enables you to fully experience your food. When your mind totally focuses on the present pleasure of eating, anxiety fades away.

Walking meditation

Look around at people walking to their various destinations. So often they rush about like hamsters on an exercise wheel, not even aware of their surroundings. Rushing people, unlike hamsters, don't enjoy the exercise — instead, their minds fill with anxious anticipations and worries. It's a small wonder that we have an epidemic of high blood pressure these days.

We have an alternative for you to consider — walking meditation. You've probably tried taking a walk sometime when you felt especially stressed. It probably helped. However, mindful walking can help you more.

Practice the following meditation while walking for five minutes, five days in a row. Then consider whether you want to make it a regular part of your life.

REMEMBER

If troubling thoughts intrude, simply notice them. Watch them like clouds floating overhead. Don't judge them. When you can, bring yourself back to the present.

TIP

Proceed with your walk as follows:

1. **Pause before you start.**

2. **Notice the feeling of air going in and out of your nose and lungs. Breathe quietly for five breaths.**

3. **Begin walking.**

4. **Notice the sensations in your leg muscles — your ankles, calves, and thighs.**

    Spend a minute or two focusing only on these muscles and how they feel.

5. **Now, feel the bottom of your feet as they strike the ground.**

    Try to notice how the heel hits first, then the foot rolls, and then you push off with the ball of your foot and toes. Concentrate on the bottom of your feet for a minute or two.

6. **Now, focus on the rhythm of your walking.**

    Feel the pace of your legs and the swing of your arms. Stay with the rhythm for a minute or two and enjoy it.

7. **Feel the air flowing into your nose and lungs. Feel yourself exhaling the air. Take notice of the rhythm of your breathing.**

    Focus on nothing else for a minute or two.

8. **Continue to take heed of your feet, muscles, rhythm, and breathing, shifting your attention from one to the other as you like.**

Enthusiasts extol the virtues of walking meditation. They claim it helps them reduce stress and become more serene. You can experiment with walking meditation in various ways. For example, try focusing on sights and sounds or focus on smells as you encounter them. Play with this strategy and develop your own approach. There's no right or wrong way to meditate.

More meditation methods

Meditation methods typically focus on something, whether it be movement, breathing, tasting, smelling, and so on. The following bullets lay out a number of the most common targets of focus:

>> **Mantra-focused meditation:** Mantras consist of words, phrases, or sounds that are repeated throughout the meditation session. Some mantras are meaningful, whereas others have no meaning at all.

- >> **Loving kindness–focused meditation:** Loving kindness meditation focuses on feelings of generosity, care, kindness, and goodwill toward yourself that you then project onto others.

- >> **Sound-focused meditation:** Sound-focused meditation may concentrate attention on sounds of nature, ocean waves, or a tone or bell.

- >> **Yoga or Tai Chi:** These are ancient forms of meditation, although many people think of them as gym classes. For meditation, these require practice and usually lessons from an expert.

This list consists of a few meditation methods you're likely to encounter. Many more exist. Consider experimenting with a few types to find one or more you like. We wish we could tell you that research strongly supports one type over another. What's particularly important is simply to choose a method and use it.

Discovering Other Meditation Resources

This chapter gave you a smorgasbord of ideas. We hope we convinced you to give meditation a try. If you're intrigued and want to find out more, you can do so in a variety of ways. Consider the following sources:

- >> **Apps:** These are simple to use, usually inexpensive, and convenient. Read the reviews carefully. Most have some kind of free trial option.

- >> **Websites:** We suggest you go for free information. You'll find lots of people wanting to charge you for various services. You don't have to spend money to learn the basics of meditation.

- >> **Classes:** These are sometimes offered at gyms, community centers, and wellness centers at low cost. They can be a great way to get started.

- >> **Books:** Lots of books are out there. One we like is *Meditation For Dummies* by Stephen Bodian (Wiley).

Buyer Beware: Meditation Myths

Unfortunately, as valuable and healthy as we believe meditation to be, there are a variety of unscrupulous characters, con artists, misguided promoters, and even some sincere believers who advocate unsupportable benefits of meditation. Meditation is rather unlikely to radically cure all ailments, make you rich, or convey magical powers to you — although you can easily find such claims. Here are a few warning signs to look out for:

>> Illogical or unrealistic promises

>> Excessive costs that escalate subtly over time

>> Celebrity endorsements

>> The necessity of frequent, lengthy training that consumes great amounts of time

>> Frequent references to a spiritual leader who has seemingly magical powers

REMEMBER

Meditation is a relatively simple, straightforward skill. It needn't cost a great deal to learn. And, it shouldn't consume your life. Realistic amounts of practice are helpful. If something doesn't feel right about a promotion, training, or product, check it out.

4

Zeroing in on Specific Worries

Chapter **13**

Emotional Preparedness During a Pandemic

n 2010, we wrote the precursor for this book. In a chapter called "Staying Healthy," we included the following paragraph:

> "Some people find that their worries about health spin out of control. They avoid crowded places. When venturing out, they wear surgical masks and carry disinfectants. Fear causes them to severely restrict their activities and interferes with their ability to enjoy life fully. These people have health anxiety."

Wow, has the world turned upside down or what? Just a decade ago, those activities seemed over the top, extreme, even pathological. Now, wearing a mask, carrying a disinfectant, and social distancing are completely reasonable, rational responses to a pandemic. It's interesting to note that the same behaviors in different circumstances can be viewed as either mentally healthy or downright neurotic.

TIP

A particularly important component of being mentally healthy involves the ability to shift behaviors when conditions change. And conditions certainly have changed!

In this chapter, we talk about adjusting to the anxiety of living through a worldwide health crisis. Since the beginning of the COVID-19 pandemic, rates of anxiety have soared throughout the world. Therefore, we provide a variety of strategies for dealing with understandable anxiety, isolation, and fear related to realistic pandemic concerns.

We share ideas about what you need to have stored in your pantry and what is excessive. We help you develop plans for deciphering conflicting messages and knowing what to believe and what to disregard. We give you ideas about accepting uncertainty and evaluating risks. Finally, we discuss the conflict between risk tolerance and value-based priorities in determining what to do.

Pushing Through Pandemic-Related Anxiety and Stress

A pandemic occurs when a wide area of the globe and a large number of people are infected by a contagious disease. Terrifying. The very thought of a pandemic frightens most people whether they normally suffer from excessive anxiety or not. However, for people who tend to be anxious, not only thinking about, but actually living through a pandemic can feel quite devastating.

If a pandemic doesn't make you stressed or anxious, you may have your head in the sand. The facts are compelling: Millions have been infected by the COVID-19 virus, and at least hundreds of thousands have already died with many more likely to come. Media stories abound concerning ways you can theoretically contract the virus including aerosol spray released by flushing a public toilet, breathing in droplets released by a stranger's sneeze or cough, or scratching your face after contact with a contaminated doorknob or countertop. It's no wonder that worries spiral out of control and people dwell on questions like:

>> What can I do to stay safe?

>> What do I need to stay alive and okay?

>> Where can I even find hand sanitizer?

>> How can I deal with all this overwhelming fear?

>> What's going to happen to me?

>> How can I get through the day?

>> How can I stand being alone?

>> How can I possibly remain 100 percent safe?

>> Who's telling the truth?

>> Will my life ever be normal again?

It's pretty easy to let your mind run wild with all the possible risks. Although there are no definitive answers to most of these questions, the following sections help you deal with anxiety and uncertainty.

Accepting emotions

One theme that shows up in various chapters of this book is that avoiding emotions only makes coping more difficult. The more desperately you try to avoid anxiety, the more likely it will thrive. During a pandemic, it's pretty normal for people to wonder, "what if?"

There are real risks. Getting the disease can be life-changing or life-threatening. People are isolated, losing their jobs, and cancelling vacations. Gyms have emptied, and many restaurants have gone out of business. So, how do you survive when day-to-day life has been upended? We see three major ways of coping with the massive stressors associated with a pandemic. Denying and wallowing make things worse, and acceptance improves daily functioning. The sections that follow describe these ways of coping.

Denying

People who deny the real risks posed by a pandemic (or any other calamity) attempt to pretend that nothing has changed. They may seek validation of their denial by finding like-minded souls on social media. Deniers may resent restrictions and public health directives. If they happen to be lucky, their denial is not challenged by the reality of getting sick themselves or having a loved one suffer. However, most people who use denial as a coping mechanism inadvertently ramp up their risk for exposure. They also feel a need to emotionally defend their denial to others. That defense can lead to feelings of anger and rage.

When the defense of denial is shattered by reality, deniers may be left with feelings of inadequacy, shame, and defeat. Alternatively, some deniers may double down when reality challenges them and work even harder to find support for their distorted views. That support may come in the form of wild conspiracy theories and/or views based on utterly irrational ideas.

Wallowing

This response consists of dwelling on all the possible and actual threats, inconveniences, losses, grief, and massive changes to lifestyle. People who respond this way have a point, and mentally healthy people will probably spend at least some time wallowing. No problem with that. It really is a pretty terrible time for many people, and everyone suffers stress and worry.

So, yes, spend some time wallowing. But in the long run, wallowing increases anxiety and depression. Thus, after a while, it's time to move on, and discover a way to accept what is.

Acceptance

After a bit of denial and wallowing, it's best for your emotional adjustment to move forward and accept reality. Those who accept take a hard look at the facts within their lives as well as in their communities. With the facts in hand, they find the best strategies for coping through problem-solving, soliciting help, and adjusting their ways of living during troubling times.

Distinguishing between useful and useless pandemic-related anxiety

Being worried during a pandemic is perfectly natural. In fact, worry can be quite useful — it may keep you from doing something unsafe or prepare you to take action. However, some worry can be useless and unproductive. Table 13-1 shows you a few examples of useful worries and actions they can lead to.

TABLE 13-1   **Useful Worries and Actions**

Useful Anxieties	Productive Actions
The supermarket is really crowded and risky on Saturday mornings when I like to go.	I need to stop going on Saturday mornings and find a time that's less crowded.
My job is still paying me, but I could lose it if this goes on too long.	I can take this time off work to learn a new skill like bookkeeping or coding. Meanwhile, I'll cut every cost I can find in my budget — bare bones!
I'm worried about inhaling the virus when I have to run a few, quick errands.	I can wear a three-layer mask and keep my distance. I could even add a face shield for more protection if I'm particularly worried about a given location.
I'm gaining weight eating so much during this isolation time. How can I lose it and stay healthy?	I need to find other things to do: I've always liked reading and jogging, so I can get back to those pleasures. And I can indulge a bit here and there. A daily menu can help too.

As Table 13-1 makes clear, it's easy to see how certain worries lead to effective problem-solving. In those cases, worries work for your benefit. However, other worries aren't so good for you. They don't as easily lead to productive actions. Examples of useless worries include

- » Will I die from this?

- » When will all this be over?

- » Will my friends or family come down with the virus?

- » What's going to happen to my retirement funds?

- » What if . . . (which leads to limitless possibilities for other worries)?

WHY PEOPLE HOARD TOILET PAPER

Perhaps you've noticed, during most disasters, toilet paper disappears quickly from the shelves, having been snapped up by anxious shoppers. You see news coverage of people pushing grocery carts stacked with enough toilet paper to last months. This behavior seems a bit strange when you consider that you can't eat toilet paper; it's substitutable with tissue, paper towels, and even wash cloths in a pinch. It's rather yucky to ponder, but toilet paper probably isn't the absolutely most critical item on an emergency list. It's probably more important to have an adequate supply of food, water, and medicine, as opposed to toilet paper.

But people hoard toilet paper. Why? Part of the reason is that toileting is associated with basic cleanliness and sanitary conditions. Unsanitary conditions are associated with risk for disease. Furthermore, toileting is one of the first behaviors toddlers are encouraged to master. Caregivers heap praise when the child is finally able to consistently poop in the toilet!

We're not suggesting people desperately shopping for toilet paper are concerned about their own toilet training. It's simply a powerful link to early learning experiences of controlling important bodily functions. So, when life seems unmanageable, there is a natural impulse to find something, anything, that will bring back some sense of control. Thus, having an ample toilet paper supply becomes a method of restraining the anxiety that comes when the world seems out of control.

If you want to buy a few extra rolls of toilet paper, have at it. But, if you feel driven and almost obsessed with "having enough," step back for a minute before you become part of the problem. Think about what's driving you to hoard. It's probably not really fear of running short on toilet paper, but fear of losing control. Focus on what you can do and getting what you truly need.

This worry list doesn't directly lead to useful actions. Instead, the questions lead to more worry and hand-wringing. That's because there are no real answers to any of them. But there are a few actions you may be able to take even on these seemingly dead-end worries. Consider

>> Taking reasonable precautions for protecting yourself and your family by following current health guidelines

>> Focusing on living the best, most meaningful life you can

>> Realizing that uncertainty is the state of life and embracing it the best you can

Gathering emergency supplies

One way to deal with pandemic-related anxiety is for all households to consider having a reasonable stockpile of supplies that exceeds day-to-day needs. Although predicting when the next disaster will come along is impossible, you can rest assured that someday, something will. The Red Cross and the U.S. Government both recommend that you have at least a three-day supply of food and water (one gallon per person per day for drinking and sanitation). In addition, the following items appear on most short-term emergency preparedness lists:

>> Face coverings for everyone over the age of two in the household

>> Prescription and nonprescription medications (anti-diarrhea, antacid, pain relievers including aspirin and ibuprofen), extra eyeglasses or contact lenses and solution

>> Hand sanitizers, soap, disinfecting wipes

>> First-aid kit with bandages, tweezers, tape, antiseptic wipes, thermometer, latex gloves, gauze

>> Flashlight with extra batteries, portable radio with weather channels (NOAA)

>> Duct tape, plastic garbage bags, can opener, wrench or pliers, whistle, fire extinguisher, multi-function tool

>> Matches or lighters

>> Pet food

>> Cash and important documents

>> Utensils, cups

>> Paper and pencil

>> Blankets, clothes, personal hygiene items

>> Oh yes, and toilet paper of course!

You may come up with additional items. Consider your family's unique needs. The important consideration is that you have these supplies within easy access and in good condition.

Please note that no list will change the basic reality that life is uncertain and that you can't prepare for every imaginable emergency. Do the best you can.

REMEMBER

Setting daily goals ✕

People around the world have had their lives changed by the pandemic. Whether you live in a large city, small town, suburb, or family farm, your life was disrupted in multiple ways. Many businesses were shut down; people were told to shelter in place, and travel was highly restricted.

Those who could, worked from home. Many others were laid off. This massive shift caused millions of people to spend most of their time at home whether working or not. And this situation naturally led to a range of powerful feelings, both positive and negative. On the positive end, some reported reduced stress because commuting was out of the picture. Others said they rediscovered the joy of reading, cooking, gardening, or watching movies.

On the negative side of the equation, many reported feeling bored, trapped, and apathetic. A large percentage of people across the globe experienced increased anxiety about money, health of self and family, careers, and relationships. The combination of apathy and anxiety is particularly problematic. That's because anxiety makes people feel awful, but apathy robs them of the motivation needed to do something about it. The more passive and unengaged you feel, the more likely you are to have anxiety.

Thus, one of the best ways to tackle anxiety is to actively engage in productive actions. That's hard to do when feeling apathetic, so we recommend starting with small steps. A daily "To-Do List" is a practical, doable start. Here are a few suggestions:

>> **Exercise:** Exercise is an effective anti-anxiety strategy. Everyone can exercise at home; you don't need a gym, as nice as that would be. No fancy equipment is required to do squats, sit-ups, push-ups, or planks. You can jog or march in place. Turn up the music. Search the internet for a variety of short, at-home workout routines. Note that activity trackers are a great way to motivate you and monitor your progress. See Chapter 11 for more information about exercise.

>> **Household chores:** Keeping an organized, clean home will lift your spirits. Some people like to schedule chores on a once-a-week basis; others prefer to break them into small chunks each day. If you have multiple people living in your house, involve them too.

>> **Maintenance:** Most homes require a bit of maintenance from time to time in addition to cleaning. If possible, choose something small such as washing a couple of windows, painting a bathroom, weeding outside for 30 minutes, trimming a bush, or patching a couple of small holes in the wall.

>> **Healthy living:** Since you're stuck cooking at home, consider developing a new habit of health-conscious meal planning and preparation. If changing your diet is too ambitious, start with one meal a week — then gradually add in another. In addition, make sure you're setting aside sufficient sleep time.

>> **Worry time:** What? Yes, if you find yourself ruminating with worrisome thoughts rambling through your head throughout the day, schedule a block of time, about 15 minutes or so, to do nothing but worry! Sounds counterintuitive, but it's not. When worry thoughts intrude, you can always tell them you've reserved a time slot for them later in the day.

>> **Entertainment:** Just because you're locked up in your home doesn't mean you can't do anything for entertainment. As annoying as it is to not have access to indoor movies, restaurants, bowling, bars, concerts, galleries, and theater, there's an array of options available on your devices. Online gaming, word games, television series (binge-watching), books, movies, and more are a click away.

WARNING

If you're a news junkie, great. You need to keep up with what's happening and the latest guidelines. However, limit your time with media. Too much media exposure is likely to increase your anxiety.

Staying connected

Numerous studies tell us that all emotional disorders are made worse by isolation from other people. And contact with others helps improve your emotional functioning. Despite obvious challenges, it's still possible to connect with others during a time of social distance. Online meetings are a start. The phone works, too. Consider forming a small group for discussing books, recipe sharing, current events, or movies. There are multiple free online platforms for holding video meetings.

TIP

If you're bored out of your mind (or even if you're not), consider contacting old friends, relatives you've lost touch with, or neighbors who may be more bored or lonely than you are! You don't have to have a long conversation in order for the connection to be meaningful. You might just say that you're thinking about them and want to make sure that they're alright. It doesn't take much to convey caring.

Figuring out Fact versus Fiction

In recent years, the term "fake news" has become commonplace in the nation's vocabulary. Fake news was historically relegated to the promotion of various political agendas. However, during the COVID-19 pandemic, fake news has also been used to influence health behavior in the public square. That is a problem — especially when people are guided to act in ways that may increase the risk of infection for themselves or others.

What makes people susceptible to fake news? There are several psychological principles that help explain this vulnerability to believing false information. People are readily influenced to come to incorrect conclusions because of a variety of *cognitive biases*. Cognitive biases refer to errors in thinking that occur in order to simplify incoming information. Here are a few that commonly occur in the discourse about public health decisions:

>> **Confirmation bias:** This bias involves the brain's tendency to pay attention to information that confirms or validates what's already believed. This bias also allows the brain to ignore what it doesn't believe. For example, if someone is determined to send her kids back to school, she's likely to seek out information about the benefits and safety of opening classrooms. At the same time, she'll discount or ignore contradictory information that advises more caution.

>> **Repetition bias:** A surprisingly powerful type of thinking bias is known as repetition bias. This bias shows up often in advertising. Have you ever wondered why marketers repeat the same ad over and over and over again? It's because the more often you're exposed to information, the more the brain finds it believable. Studies have shown this effect to occur even when the initial information was not believed by the recipients. Regarding COVID-19, you no doubt have heard repeated bombardment of messaging around the idea that "it's all under control." Repetition bias is primitive and simplistic, but shockingly effective at distorting reality.

>> **Narrative bias:** The brain likes stories, and they're easy to remember. Almost any message you want to convey will be easier to sell if it's wrapped in an interesting or compelling story. For example, when you hear that 200,000 people have died from COVID-19, you probably feel bad. However, if you hear about a young mother who dies leaving four children behind or a beloved emergency room doctor who died from Covid, which he caught caring for his patients, you're likely to feel much stronger emotions. You'll also recall these examples more easily and vividly.

>> **Cognitive dissonance:** Cognitive dissonance occurs when people have a belief and a behavior that are contradictory to each other. For example, imagine a graduating senior has planned a large graduation party but also has the belief that large crowds increase the risks of an infection. The student

will be motivated to reconcile the contradictory behavior and thought by changing one of them. Thus, the student may justify the party by adopting a less malignant view of the risks involved, or alternatively, may decide to cancel the party. Note that the motivation is to simplify a seeming contradiction as opposed to careful consideration of evidence and facts.

>> **Correlation as causation bias:** This bias involves the tendency to causally link two sequential events. In other words, when A occurs first, followed by B, it's easy to assume that A caused B. For example, imagine someone goes to the grocery store wearing a mask and frequently using hand sanitizer. The next day, he spikes a fever and gets tested — with a positive COVID-19 result. He concludes that the grocery store is where he picked up the infection. However, he also had multiple contacts with family members at a backyard barbeque the week before. The biased response is to assume the grocery store was the source, whereas the reality is that the source is very much unknown.

It's important to realize just how powerfully cognitive biases influence everyone's thinking processes. It's not easy to take the time to sort through evidence and withhold judgment until all the data has been considered and sifted. Here are some questions to ask yourself when you're presented with possibly exaggerated or erroneous information:

>> What evidence is this story based on?

>> Can I think of any counter examples?

>> Do I see inconsistencies in the message?

>> Am I just hearing what I expect to hear?

>> Are there missing pieces to the puzzle?

>> Am I dismissing this message because I'd have to change my mind?

>> Am I tempted to believe this because I've heard it so much?

>> Is there proof that A caused B, or could something else be responsible? If so, which is more likely?

>> Are my emotions being provoked with a compelling story?

>> Do the facts line up to support what's being said?

>> What, if anything, would convince me that this message is false?

WARNING

Cognitive biases affect everyone's thinking and judgment. Indeed, they help you make decisions more quickly, although at some cost to accuracy. However, when it comes to issues like public health and pandemics, you want to minimize the influence of bias, and adhere as closely as you can to facts, evidence, and science.

Is this the end of the world?

The world, the future, and life itself is fraught with uncertainty. That's an undeniable fact. However, the human brain is hardwired to greatly prefer certainty over uncertainty. People readily prepare for the certain. The uncertain future is unknowable and therefore, provides a fertile field for anxiety to flourish.

For example, when terminally ill patients have an idea of when they might die, they often report a sense of relief. They make plans, say goodbye to loved ones, and emotionally prepare. Everyone knows that there is an end date to life, but not knowing when provokes increased anxiety.

The unknown risks of a pandemic to any particular person increases everyone's fears. You know that there are dangers, but you don't know when or if you will encounter them. The uncertainty causes distress.

However, paradoxically, you need to confront the reality of uncertainty in life in order to combat the distress of the unknowable. This radical acceptance of the unacceptable helps you discover your inner strength. The alternative is to avoid acceptance of uncertainty by continuing the unwinnable struggle. Letting go of the need to control and find certainty allows you to let go of worry.

Is it safe to leave your house?

When events like a pandemic occur, there are many individual decisions to be made. For example:

>> Is it safe to go to an indoor restaurant?

>> Is it safe to shop for groceries, and if so, how?

>> When can I see my friends?

>> Can I go on a vacation?

>> Can I visit my family?

>> Is it safe to fly, and what do I need to do to protect myself?

>> Should I send my kids back to school?

There are no absolute answers to these questions and no positive certainty. Life is not totally safe, and public health crises increase the risks. Your best sources for making decisions come from mainstream public health professionals, disease experts, and scientists. They are able to give you general, best predictions based on evidence. However, risks remain, and personal values also enter into the equation.

For example, you may not be willing to go to an inside restaurant when it's deemed reasonably safe to do so. Dining in a restaurant is probably not that important to you. But you may decide to attend a protest with a large crowd even if it poses similar risks. That's because your value system helps you determine that the risk of possible infection is worth making because of your strong commitment to the cause.

Similarly, you may decide that travel to visit a close family member is important enough to consider flying once risks moderate a little. These individual decisions are based on the inevitable tension between science and deeply held personal values.

Unfortunately, some people fail to factor in the value of not harming others as opposed to doing what they personally want. For example, some choose not to wear masks because of a belief in "personal freedom"; others host large, uncontrolled gatherings that raise the risks of an outbreak. These seemingly personal decisions can cause harm to first responders, healthcare workers, and innocent bystanders.

It's difficult to balance concepts like freedom versus responsibility. When you have personal freedom, it's important to respect the freedom of others to live healthy lives. Making choices during a public health crisis that puts others at risk inevitably takes away that freedom.

Chapter **14**

Facing a Career Crisis and Financial Woes

P eople worry about money — a lot. They obsess over their 401(k) accounts, savings, salaries, home values, and promotions. More basic needs underlie these concerns — worries about job loss, foreclosures, and the ability to meet essential life needs such as food, clothing, healthcare, and shelter. Although people are clearly more important than money, everyone needs a certain amount of income for survival.

In this chapter, we tackle money concerns head-on. We do so with a keen awareness of the seriousness of financial worries. In other words, we don't take a glib, *don't worry, be happy* approach to these issues. And we don't claim to be financial experts; after all, we're psychologists. So this chapter is not a prescription for getting rich fast and retiring early. It's a guide to what steps you can take to better handle your anxiety and worry over your career and financial challenges.

First, we take a hard-nosed look at job worries. Then, we help you make a realistic appraisal of what you have and don't have. We also guide you through an exercise that explores your true needs as separate from your mere desires and wishes. Finally, we ask you to commit to a new, long-term financial strategy designed to minimize your financial worries.

Meeting Job Worries Head-On

If you worry about losing your job, you're in good company. Like it or not, economic recessions occur every so many years and often result in millions of people losing their jobs. And one can ever know for certain which careers will become the most vulnerable in the next recession. Thus, at one time, working for a major car manufacturer was seen as one of the most secure jobs you could have.

Technology has produced huge numbers of jobs in some areas while wiping out or depleting opportunities for many jobs such as travel agents, telephone operators, and bank tellers. Further into the future, technological advances are likely to greatly impact the jobs of people who drive for a living as autonomous vehicles come into widespread use. Online shopping may eventually eliminate most brick-and-mortar stores as well as the jobs of clerks who run the cash registers.

The recent pandemic caused the loss of millions of jobs. And for most of those who've held on to jobs, salary increases have stalled and opportunities for advancement have vanished, at least for the short run. If you're faced with possible job loss, anxiety is a perfectly understandable emotion. Of course, you worry! This section gives you a few tools for dealing with these worries.

Shoring up your resume

One way to decrease your worries about jobs is to maximize your marketability. Even if you're currently working, it's a good idea to have a world-class resume. You can easily find sample resumes and tips for writing them online. Or consider reading *Resumes For Dummies* by Laura DeCarlo (Wiley). If you're out of work, check out the book from your local library.

Keeping your resume up-to-date sounds simple, right? But it's not necessarily so. Many people find resume-writing highly anxiety-arousing. And when people have anxiety, they tend to avoid what makes them anxious. So, if you're like many people, you may find yourself procrastinating or avoiding the task.

TIP

We have some suggestions:

>> **Get help.** If you've lost your job, state unemployment offices and local community colleges offer training on writing resumes.

>> **Break the task into small steps.** For example, vow to write out your educational background during the first session. The next day, write out your job descriptions.

>> **Show your resume to a few friends or colleagues for feedback.** Or, if you're working with an employment agency, someone there can likely give you pointers.

>> **Know that avoiding this task will likely increase your anxiety rather than make you feel better.** The only way to get through that anxiety is to face your fear by going right at it and tackling the task in spite of your anxiety.

Employers often spend no more than ten seconds reviewing each individual resume. Make sure yours is short, visually appealing, and highlights your best strengths. You can't afford to have any misspellings or grammatical errors.

If your resume review reveals a lack of skills, you may want to consider acquiring new skills, either on your own or through a local training facility, community college, or university. See the "Considering careers with stability" section later in the chapter for fields that generally offer relatively steady employment.

Finding flexibility in your career view

Whether you lose a job because of layoffs, can't find a job in your own field, or simply choose to leave a job, a psychological trait known as flexibility can improve your ability to handle the challenge of change. Flexible people adapt to new situations. When stuck, they look for alternatives. They take action to improve their situation.

So, why is flexibility so important for handling job worries? According to the U.S. Department of Labor, an average worker holds 11.7 jobs between the ages of 18 and 48. Obviously, there's a wide range — some people never have more than 1 or 2 jobs and others have 20. The message is that very few people stay with one company for a lifetime of work. In addition, many people switch careers — some by choice (like after obtaining additional training) and others by accident (such as losing a job in one field and taking a job in another field).

Inflexible people often become angry when faced with job frustrations. Instead of acting, they react with anger at how unfair life has been for them. Inflexible people stick to old choices, don't take advantage of new opportunities, and seem stubborn and stuck.

To improve *physical* flexibility, you start with small stretches and gradually bend more. If a move is too painful, you back down. You try to achieve balance by stretching both the right and left sides of your body. Gradually, your flexibility improves.

Mental flexibility involves the same principles — gradual steps, balance, and backing off when things become too painful. Mental flexibility involves being able to see reality from different perspectives. For example, in a job interview, a person with mental flexibility would try to put himself in the shoes of the person doing the interview. Or in negotiations, a flexible person would take the time to consider the perspectives of all involved.

Mental flexibility accepts change as inevitable and expected. Such flexibility requires openness to new experiences and the understanding that most of the time, truth is unknowable. Finally, flexible people understand that in order to learn, they must listen.

Armed with a more flexible attitude, you can handle the stress and anxiety of job loss and other changes by considering all your options and alternatives. This attitude may enable you to see possibilities you wouldn't see otherwise. And your efforts will more likely result in success.

When writing your resume (see the preceding section), use flexible thinking. Look at your past jobs and consider what skills, attributes, and characteristics you brought to the table above and beyond those that are obvious from your job titles — highlight these skills on your resume. And when you interview, mention the connection between the skills you've acquired and how you can use them to advantage in your new company, instead of focusing on the past.

Considering careers with stability

You'll worry less if your career path stands on a concrete foundation rather than one made of sand. If you're underemployed or unemployed, consider updating your skills or changing your career path to one that has more stability. Get more training and education. If figuring out how to pay for classes is a concern, most postsecondary schools have student loans, grants, or other ways to help pay for their programs. Better yet, consider a work-study program if offered. You'll get valuable experience and possibly develop connections that could pay off with a job offer when your studies are complete.

It's never too late to go back to school. Consider taking one class at a time. Also, look into online courses from accredited schools. These classes can be especially convenient for some people.

Think about how many years you have left to work. Wouldn't you prefer to be doing something you like? Here are a few areas considered to be *relatively* stable in these unstable times:

>> **Healthcare:** Almost all areas of healthcare will see growth over the next few decades. In addition to professionals like nurses, doctors, pharmacists, physical therapists, occupational therapists, and dentists, others, such as home healthcare workers, medical technologists, and healthcare case managers, will be in greater demand.

>> **Technical jobs:** As more of life migrates online, technical engineers, information security analysts, computer coders, data-based administrators, and market researchers will be needed.

>> **Education:** As the baby boomers retire from teaching, the education system will see many openings. Areas of need continue to exist in math, science, and bilingual education. College instructors and professors will also be needed in greater numbers.

>> **Law enforcement and security:** Needs for police officers, correction officers, and security personnel are likely to increase in years to come. Many of those working in this field are slated for retirement in the coming decade or so.

>> **Green jobs:** Assuming you've heard or read a news report in the last few years, you know that there has been a cry for increasing energy independence and minimizing the harmful impact humans have on the environment. Thus, this emphasis will call for a vast pool of workers trained in areas such as engineering, chemistry, physics, hydrology, and ecology, as well as technological expertise in almost every imaginable type of alternative energy. These jobs will be available for both those with advanced degrees and those with manufacturing and technical skills. Many community colleges offer training in these emerging industries.

WARNING

No career path comes with a guarantee of stability. Accept that what's stable at one time could become less so later. Remember, you need to be flexible.

TIP

Traditionally used by school guidance and vocational counselors, the *Occupational Outlook Handbook* is available for free at www.bls.gov/ooh/. It contains a comprehensive listing of jobs, educational requirements, job conditions, and salaries. The U.S. Bureau of Labor Statistics updates this book frequently. Also, check out the Dictionary of Occupational Titles available at www.occupationalinfo.org for more ideas. Use it to broaden your list of possibilities. Again, be flexible!

Keeping the right focus

Anxiety, fear, and dread can easily overwhelm you if you let them. When faced with the possibility of job or income loss, people fill their minds with images of living on the streets or dying of hunger. Such a scenario is indeed awful, and it occasionally happens. But you can do much to prevent this outcome, and it occurs a very small fraction of the time compared to the amount of time that people spend dwelling on this worry.

If you worry about losing your job or you find yourself unemployed, you have a new job. That new job is to cut your expenses to the bone (we give you some guidance on making these cuts in the "Tallying up your financial balance sheet" section later in the chapter). Cutting expenses helps you even if you haven't yet lost your job, because it helps you hold out longer if you do lose your income. After you've reduced the amount of money you're spending, your next step is to maximize your ability to find a new job (more on that in the "Knowing your personal assets and liabilities" section).

Other strategies, such as applying for unemployment, getting help from families, and applying for food stamps, should all be considered. But go to your state unemployment office for the nuts and bolts of that kind of advice. From a psychological perspective, we suggest the following:

>> Focus on the present, taking one day at a time.

>> Take care of your physical body by eating right and exercising to help your mind.

>> Stay connected with friends and family — support helps!

>> Consider going to a support group for job seekers — find one through the internet or your local newspaper.

>> Realize that negative predictions and worrying about possible future calamities never prevented a single catastrophe.

Taking Stock of Your Resources

Personal resources include financial and psychological assets and liabilities. *Assets* are the money or skills that you have that are of great value; *liabilities* are the money you owe or the skills that you need to gain. Both play a critical role in your adjustment to setbacks and stress. The following sections outline some of the things that can help maximize your assets and minimize your liabilities.

Tallying up your financial balance sheet

Most lenders such as mortgage companies, banks, or car dealers require customers to fill out loan applications. A standard <u>loan</u> application includes a description of the purpose of the loan and information about the borrowers. The application often asks about money coming in each month as well as monthly expenses. Applicants are also asked to list all their assets and liabilities. A net worth is calculated by subtracting the liabilities from the assets.

You don't have to apply for a loan to organize your assets. We suggest that you review your income, expenses, assets, and liabilities whether or not you want to borrow money. That way you can see just what you have now. Make a list for each of the four categories; the result is called your *balance sheet.*

REMEMBER

When you think about your assets, include everything — grandma's silver, coin collections, and other prized possessions. You may not want to sell them, but you always know you could if things got really bad.

After you know your income, expenses, assets, and liabilities, take a moment to think about them. Can you find ways to improve your balance sheet? We suggest that you carefully review your expenses. All too often, people make the mistake of assuming they *need* far more than they really do. Like the environment calls for reducing your carbon footprint, consider reducing your financial footprint. It will be good for the environment (less stuff to manufacture) and particularly good for your wallet.

In order to get started, ponder the answers to these questions:

>> How could I entertain myself without 150 TV stations? People used to get by on one to three channels when TV first showed up on the scene. You don't have to pare back that far to save money. Comb through your monthly subscription services, and only keep the ones that are fairly priced and that you use frequently. Many people hold onto subscriptions they rarely use.

>> How many outfits do I really wear regularly, and how few could I get by on? Try sticking to solid colors of good quality clothing. Shop thrift stores for gently used outfits — you can find designer outfits if you shop carefully. And you can get by with much less variety. It's unlikely people will notice.

>> Can I cut out unnecessary coffee, lunches, and dinners out? You can cut back substantially here. Try getting by on once-a-month special meals from a restaurant (take-out if conditions require).

>> Can I drink more water and less soda and alcohol? Buy a few lemons or limes to add more flavor. It's healthier and cheaper.

>> How can I cut my use of the car by walking, biking, or using public transportation? You can keep your car longer — they go much farther than they used to. That will save you thousands of dollars.

>> How much could I save by checking books out of the library instead of purchasing them? Most libraries have an extensive selection of e-books in addition to hard-copy books.

>> How can I cut my energy use and save money? If you own your house, carefully do the math to see if solar energy pays off — don't just trust the salesperson.

>> Can I stop smoking? Smoking literally burns money and negatively impacts your health — costing you much more. Consider buying a copy of our book *Quitting Smoking & Vaping For Dummies* (Wiley).

>> How can I spend less on the gym? First, shop around. Gyms offer a wide range of prices and services. And, if you're serious about saving money, you can exercise for free by walking or jogging in the park. You can also find great, short exercise routines online.

>> Can I stop spending money to impress other people? Others pay less attention to your car, home, clothes, and your professionally styled hair than you think. But even if they do, does their opinion truly matter?

Multiple research studies have found what most people have trouble believing: Your income has a very small relationship to how happy you are. Many people find that once they start cutting expenses, they're amazed at how much they can save without sacrificing their emotional well-being. In fact, they often report feeling less stressed. Some even say that the saving process feels like fun when they get going.

Knowing your personal assets and liabilities

Although you want to assess your financial strengths first when facing the possibility of a job loss, it's also helpful to analyze your personal strengths and attributes. Start by asking yourself the following questions:

>> Am I willing to learn new skills?

>> Do I get along well with other people?

>> Am I persistent?

>> Do I get to work on time?

>> Do I finish projects on time?

>> Do I accept feedback and criticism without becoming defensive?

>> Am I a good team player?

» Do I refrain from unnecessary gossiping?

» Do I keep my personal life separate from my professional life?

» Am I self-motivated?

» Am I good at keeping my cool under stress?

» Am I creative, and can I think outside the box?

In an interview, be prepared to talk about any of the preceding questions that you feel you can answer affirmatively; these represent your assets. If your answers to any of the questions are negative, they may represent areas for personal development. Look for ways to improve in those areas to turn your liabilities into assets.

TIP

After writing out your answers to the preceding list of questions, write down as many of your personal strengths as you can think of. Consider including examples from previous jobs that illustrate these strengths. Then list your weaker areas. The result gives you a sense of your job-related, psychological net worth.

Committing to a New Game Plan

You can reduce the amount of energy you spend worrying about jobs and money if you commit yourself to making some changes. In addition to the ideas in the previous sections, we suggest you develop a game plan for your money and your career. We recommend that you consider both short- and long-term goals. Earlier sections prepare you for what's next — where the rubber meets the road.

Setting short-term goals

You'll never get where you want to go unless you have a map. Lots of people go through their entire lives without ever thinking about what they want to accomplish. Look at your money and career, and ponder what you really want to achieve in the next couple of years.

Considering short-term career goals

Take a vocational interest inventory at your local community college. Write down the job skills that you already possess. Brainstorm job possibilities that can make use of your personal strengths and interests. Make a list of these job possibilities and, assuming you've updated your resume, prepare to market yourself.

TIP

Prior to putting in applications, we recommend that you practice interviewing with your friends or a vocational counselor or therapist. Practice until your anxiety comes down — and it will if you practice enough.

When you've got a polished resume and you're ready to face an interviewer, you need to find a job. Don't just rely on sending out resumes to jobs listed on the internet. In addition to those sources, consider

TIP

» Making a list of employers that sound interesting to work for. Investigate the companies through searches and sign up for updates on employment search engines — often free to applicants.

» Preparing a series of questions relevant to the company you're interested in. For example, "Are there opportunities for advancement?" "What training opportunities exist in the company?" "Is it possible to work from home?"

» Calling people you used to work or go to school with — in other words, networking.

» Asking family and friends — more networking.

» Working for a temporary agency — those jobs often become permanent.

TIP

If all else fails and you really need some income, consider a job from the gig economy (a market of short-term contracts and freelance work) such as driving or delivery services. The advantages are that these jobs are easy to get and money transfers to your account quickly. Note that important disadvantages include a lack of benefits and the fact that expenses generally fall on the worker. The pay often looks better than it is if you calculate the costs carefully. Nonetheless, sometimes you need the cash these jobs provide.

Getting your money plans started

Money flows like water. If you stop spending it in one area, it flows around that area just to be spent somewhere else. The only way to save it is to channel your money carefully into a reservoir or holding tank. Yes, we're talking about saving.

Because this isn't an investment book, we're not going to suggest specific types of investments. Rather, the purpose of this book is to help you understand and deal with anxiety. So if you're anxious about money, you'll have less anxiety if you have more money saved. And it doesn't matter much where you put it — money adds up even in a savings account with zero percent interest.

So start now. Begin with what you have and build slowly. Continually increase your contributions to your savings as soon as you can. You may just surprise yourself.

Planning for the long haul

Not too many years ago, people worked for the same company for a lifetime and looked forward to a retirement of fishing and golf. More often than not, nowadays that dream is just that — a dream that won't ever find fulfillment, at least as it was originally envisioned. Many jobs have evaporated, a surprising number of pension plans have gone belly up, and some IRA and 401(k) types of accounts have failed to meet expectations.

Is this state of affairs a cause for despair and hopelessness? We don't think so. Sure, you're right to feel concerned and maybe even disappointed that you may not be able to retire when you want or live the retirement lifestyle that you once expected. But the trait of flexibility we talk about earlier in this chapter applies here, too. You should know that research reported in the *Journal of Occupational Health Psychology* actually found that people who work part time instead of completely retiring are healthier both physically and mentally. This finding held up even when controlling for variables like age, education, and wealth.

So, consider that the goal of complete retirement may not even be especially good for you! You don't have to make as much as you did prior to semi-retiring or work as many hours. That's because part-time work can go a long way toward stretching whatever retirement account dollars you already have. Consider looking for an encore career that gives you more satisfaction and meaning than just money. Or try something brand new that comes with less stress but connects you with people. It's a whole lot easier to go to work if you're having fun. At this time in your life, your job doesn't need to build your ego or impress other people.

Finally, try to realize that a certain amount of uncertainty is certain! In other words, life and investments will always take unexpected twists and turns. You can't avoid setbacks, but you can recover. In the long haul, markets, economies, and people inevitably rise and fall.

Chapter **15**

Keeping Steady When the World Is Shaking

P erhaps you think that you're a rational person. If so, you probably believe that the fears that make you the most anxious are the things that pose the greatest risk to you — after all, that would be the most rational perspective, wouldn't it? But that's not how the mind works. People focus and dwell on worries that grab their attention, not those that are most likely to happen.

News media, inadvertently or otherwise, often exacerbate the problem. When natural disasters hit, news helicopters take off like a flock of geese startled by a shotgun blast. Television screens fill with images of horror, pain, suffering, and death. Reporters seemingly thrive on interviews with grief-stricken victims and run their tales of woe repeatedly for days at a time. No wonder many people spend lots of time worrying about natural disasters.

On the other hand, perhaps you have a variety of anxieties and worries, but natural disasters aren't something that bother you. If so, you can feel free to skip this chapter — unless you're just curious about the subject.

In this chapter, we help you sort through such fears and worries. We help you see that you may be spending lots of time on issues of low risk and/or things you really can't do anything about. We also discuss how to look at your personal risks. Sometimes, worrying about natural disasters is realistic if you live in certain high-risk areas. In those cases, we suggest ways to manage such risks from a practical as well as emotional standpoint. We conclude with ideas about what you can do to cope actively rather than passively by working to improve the world and the lives of others when they encounter natural disasters.

Assessing Your Risks

Because images of natural disasters vividly stream from screens within minutes of their occurrence, keeping a realistic perspective on how much risk they really pose to you is often difficult. In the next couple of sections, we briefly review the types of natural disasters in the world and the frequency with which they occur. We also help you understand your true risks for encountering a natural disaster.

Looking at the likelihood of dying from a natural disaster

You've certainly heard the eternal question about when a tree falls in a forest — if no one is there to hear it, does it make a sound? Natural disasters are sort of like that tree. Are calamitous events truly calamitous if no one is around when they occur? Maybe not.

However, plenty of disasters hurt people — often in significant numbers — when they occur. Disasters can also lead to financial, environmental, and emotional distress or loss. The following list represents some of the most common natural disasters that people worry about:

>> **Avalanches** are sudden snow slides that break loose and pummel or bury anything in their path. They kill about 150 people per year. Most avalanches occur after a winter storm. The risk of dying in an avalanche can be put in perspective by knowing that the world population now stands at about 7.8 billion and counting.

>> **Earthquakes** occur thousands of times every day. The vast majority of these quakes are minor and unnoticeable on the earth's surface. From time to time, however, earthquakes unleash a powerful explosion of pent-up energy sending huge, destructive seismic waves across a broad area. On average, about 10,000 people die in earthquakes each year. Most die in collapsed buildings, but earthquake-triggered landslides, fires, and floods also claim lives.

>> **Fires,** whether in forests, houses, or buildings, kill more people than most natural disasters. The U.S. Fire Administration claims that the United States' rate of fire deaths is among the highest in the industrialized world with about 3,500 deaths a year. Worldwide, the World Health Organization reports about 180,000 deaths from fire a year.

>> **Floods** occur when large volumes of water submerge land, houses, buildings, and people. They often result from extreme weather such as hurricanes or torrential downpours. Floods also occur when dams and other barriers break. The overall risk of dying from floods has declined due to improved warning systems and knowledge about where they're likely to occur. There are concerns about increased risk of flooding due to global warming; however, the number of people who die from floods in the United States is about 100 a year.

>> **Hurricanes** emerge from some tropical storms and generate wind speeds of 75 to over 150 miles an hour. Most of those who die from hurricanes die from flooding (see the preceding item in this list).

Have we got you worried? Consider that this list pales in comparison to all the possible natural disasters. Perhaps you can't readily think of other disasters, but here's a partial list for you to worry about:

>> Asteroids

>> Blizzards and extreme cold

>> Dust storms

>> Falling junk from outer space

>> Fire tornados

>> Gamma ray bursts (massive electromagnetic explosions in galaxies that have even been speculated as having the potential to someday cause mass extinctions on earth!)

>> Hailstorms

>> Heat waves

>> Lightning

>> Limnic eruptions (a huge eruption of carbon dioxide from deep lakes that can suffocate livestock and people in the area)

>> Mudslides

» Tornados

» Tsunamis

» Volcanic eruptions

You get the idea. Possibilities abound. But your overall risk of death from any particular natural disaster is far lower than death by your own hand or accidental death — both of which *most* people worry much less about than natural disasters. On the other hand, your risk of death from natural disasters may be far greater than most people's. We tell you how to determine that risk next.

Tabulating your personal risks

The lists in the preceding section include the most common natural disasters (and obviously a number that aren't so common). But you probably don't have to worry too much about them happening to you unless you live in an area plagued by them. However, you never know when something may erupt. So, make a list of your personal risk factors. Do you live, work, travel, or play in areas that may be subject to a natural disaster?

For example, people who live in certain areas of California choose the wonderful weather over the risk of living in earthquake, fire, and mudslide risk zones. And if you go helicopter skiing frequently, you darn well better know about what triggers avalanches. So a given individual may have a much greater risk of being harmed or killed by natural disasters than the average person. If that risk applies to you, you want to take extra precautions.

TIP

If you don't know your risks, try using a search engine on the internet to find out. After all, you don't want to live in denial any more than you want to obsess about risks that are greater in your mind than in reality.

For example, we live in landlocked New Mexico and usually don't even think about natural disasters. Every once in a while, a weather system in the Pacific causes it to rain like crazy here, and we get a few flooded streets and arroyos (you might call them drainage ditches). In some areas of the state, forest fires present some risk. In addition, if you look out our home's window, you can see some dusty old volcanoes that were active about 100,000 years ago. We don't worry too much about those either.

But just to make sure, we entered "New Mexico and volcanoes" into our browser, and, much to our surprise, we found out that our state is known as the "volcano state." Furthermore, we sit on a large continental rift and live on top of large veins of hot lava. The time frame listed for another eruption was listed as "geologically soon." Oh no! What should we do? We better read up on emergency preparation for volcanos. Or not.

Assessing risks from climate change

Climate change isn't exactly a natural disaster because it's largely caused by humans. However, observable changes in the climate are causing disturbing environmental changes, many of which in turn increase risks of other disasters. Global climate change has caused rising temperatures that have resulted in rapidly melting glaciers, reductions of soil moisture, erosion, and a rise in sea levels. These temperature rises have already had devastating consequences in areas that lack adequate air conditioning. Of additional concern have been increases in insect outbreaks, droughts, and wildfires.

Hurricanes have become more frequent and destructive as well. Weather has become more unpredictable with increased incidence of heavy downpours and floods. Economic costs include escalating rates for homeowner, flood, and fire insurance. In some higher-risk areas, insurance companies refuse to issue policies.

As you can guess, calculating your personal risk from climate change is rather tricky. But it's likely that the entire world's population will be adversely affected.

CORONAVIRUS AND AIR POLLUTION

Air pollution, even small amounts, increases the risk of death from COVID-19. A Harvard University study looked at over 3,000 counties in the United States and found that increases in pollution resulted in more deaths. In addition, previous studies have found that air pollution increases people's risk for lung cancer, strokes, heart attacks, and chronic obstructive pulmonary disease (COPD). Unfortunately, a disproportionate percentage of Blacks and people of color live in areas with high rates of air pollution, which may contribute to their higher risk of dying from COVID-19.

Preparing a Plan for Realistic Worries

You can never prepare for every imaginable crisis. Rather, it's important to assess which risks have a *realistic* chance of happening. Then, prepare for those in proportion to the risks they pose, as best you can.

TIP

Probably the most important piece of advice we can give you is this: During times of crisis, listen to public service announcements and directives — and follow them. In addition, we suggest you ponder the following questions in advance of *any* calamity:

>> Have I become educated about the specific risks in my area?

>> If I live in a place in which natural disasters occur, have I made reasonable preparations?

>> Do I know the emergency evacuation route for my area?

>> If a disaster appears imminent, do I have a full tank of gas?

>> Do I have supplies on hand, such as flashlights, warm clothing, extra batteries, at least a three-day stockpile of food and water, and a battery-powered radio?

>> Do I have a first-aid kit?

>> Do I have a plan if an emergency occurs?

>> Do I have an emergency stash of cash?

>> Do I have my important documents saved in a safety deposit box or fireproof safe?

>> Do I know how to use a fire extinguisher, and do I have a fully charged extinguisher?

>> Do I know how to shut off utilities in the event of a disaster?

>> Do I know what I would take with me in case I need to evacuate?

>> Do I have a plan in place to communicate with my family?

>> Do I have a way to protect my pets?

TIP

After you've gone through the list of questions, take any actions that seem necessary and reasonable. Then stop worrying; you've done all you can do.

Note the first question on our list is: *Have I become educated about the specific risks in my area?* Thus, we searched the internet to find out what to do in case of a volcano eruption. Well, the first idea is to get out of the way. If we do happen to be stuck in the house, we should close the doors, windows, and block the chimneys to keep ash out. If we go outside to watch, we should hold a damp cloth over our mouths to help us breathe. Also, we found out that hot lava and ash are heavy and should be brushed off of our roof if much lands on it. On the other hand, sometimes volcanoes blow out chunks of lava the size of a house, so sweeping it off may be difficult. Dang.

Nevertheless, we're not planning to spend a whole lot of time on preparing for this eventuality, nor do we figure on worrying a lot about it. But after writing this chapter, we did realize it wouldn't be a bad idea to check on the state of our fire extinguisher in case any of that lava lands on our backyard or house.

REMEMBER

No matter how well you prepare, you can't prevent all calamities. Make *reasonable* efforts, and get on with your life. You can never eliminate all uncertainty from life.

Nonetheless, if you find yourself still worrying after having done all you realistically should to plan for disasters, read the next section.

FINDING THE SILVER LINING IN ADVERSITY

Unexpected things happen even if you take precautions. The following account of a couple on a honeymoon illustrates an unexpected encounter with a natural disaster.

Sandy and Brice leave for their tropical honeymoon in November, carefully avoiding the peak of hurricane season. The newlyweds are exhausted from the wedding and look forward to a relaxing beach vacation. As promised, the resort is beautiful and the beaches pristine. After the first day of lounging on the beach, they return to their room. They're surprised to see a note lying on their bed.

"The management regrets to inform you that there will be a severe tropical storm in the area. Please be advised that you will be required to evacuate by bus to a safe area. Please bring your belongings, a blanket, and a pillow. We will be leaving from the lobby of the hotel in two hours."

The buses take about 50 guests and hotel staff to a shabby school about 30 minutes away. The humidity is high, and the school smells like mold. The staff tells the guests that the air-conditioning in the school doesn't work very well, but they will try to keep everyone comfortable. Cots are set up in a large room that serves as a cafeteria and gymnasium.

(continued)

(continued)

Sandy and Brice try to keep a positive attitude, and the hotel staff seems very well organized. The first meal consists of a cold chicken salad, salsa, and chips. The hotel provides cans of beer and soda. A few of the quests start singing campfire songs, and the group remains festive. However, after a few hours, the rain picks up. Then the electricity goes off. The mood of the refugees grows darker with the darkening sky. Hours pass, and the sounds of wind, rain, and thunder are interrupted by loud crashes. People huddle together; some cry; others pray. A few exhausted children sleep.

By morning, the intensity of the storm lessens. But the people are told that it's not yet safe to return to the beach area and that the airports are closed. Brice tells a staff member that he must get in touch with his family. The staff member tells him that communication is impossible. They serve cold hard rolls and canned juice for breakfast. Staff inform them that water is getting scarce and that they must ration it. As the day wears on, anger and irritability rise. Some people get sick. The smell gets worse and worse. The third and fourth days pose almost unbearable challenges from the lack of electricity, food, water, and sanitary conditions.

Finally, the buses come back and the tourists are returned to a devastated hotel. Windows are shattered, and the halls are flooded. Sandy and Brice can barely walk, having suffered from food poisoning. Yet they feel lucky to be alive.

Sandy and Brice realize that even when you try your best to avoid risks, bad things happen. In looking back, they believe they gained maturity and closeness from the adversity. Their new marriage flourishes. And they face the coming years with greater acceptance of uncertainty and appreciation for every day of their lives.

Imagining and Dealing with the Worst

Hopefully, you've looked at how realistic your worries about natural disasters are, and you've done what you can do to plan. Nevertheless, you may find yourself worrying more than you'd like to.

Our first recommendation is to carefully read Chapters 5, 6, and 7 to understand how your feelings, thoughts, and beliefs influence your anxiety. Then, you can apply that information to your worries about natural disasters. The following sections show you how to make that application to this issue.

TIP

If you or someone you care about does experience a natural disaster, you'll probably feel increased anxiety and distress. If your distress is mild, Chapters 5, 6, and 7 may help you deal with it. If distress is severe and continues, please consider seeing a mental health professional.

Rethinking uncertainty and anxiety

The anxious mind tries in vain to eliminate all uncertainty from life. Unfortunately, living a life without a reasonable degree of uncertainty would result in more misery than you think. Consider the following list of risks, many of which you probably take every day. Imagine trying to live life without any of these risks at all.

>> Leaving your house

>> Driving your car

>> Breathing without a mask (unless a pandemic is active)

>> Eating food that hasn't been boiled

>> Opening your mail (it could have anthrax in it)

>> Going shopping

>> Walking across a street

>> Riding a bike

>> Taking a shower (poses a significant risk of falls)

Of course, we realize that if you suffer from significant anxiety, you probably do try to avoid at least a few of these risks. But you're taking many such chances regularly.

TIP

Even if you wear a mask and decontaminate every surface you touch, you can't prevent contact with all germs, natural disasters, or accidents. Even though you may think otherwise, *acceptance* of risk and uncertainty paradoxically helps anxiety abate.

Rethinking your ability to cope

Most people with anxiety disorders gravely underestimate their ability to cope in the face of unexpected challenges. They see themselves as easily overwhelmed and lacking either the will, skills, or resources to deal with adversity. For example, they say to themselves, "I couldn't stand that," "I can't take it," or "I'd fall apart if that happened to me!" Yet when they actually encounter what they fear, inevitably, they do cope.

TIP

In Chapter 6, we provide a list of five questions for helping you deal with some pretty difficult worst-case scenarios. We suggest answering these questions for your fears of natural disasters. First, we show you the questions, and then we illustrate their use with an example.

>> Have I ever dealt with anything like this in the past?

>> How much will this affect my life a year from now?

>> Do I know people who've coped with something like this, and how did they do it?

>> Do I know anyone I could turn to for help or support?

>> Can I think of a creative new possibility that could result from this challenge?

In the next example, a resident of Southern California attempts to answer the coping questions to help her deal with her fear of earthquakes.

Lynne moves from London to San Diego to take an academic position at the University of California. She loves her new job and the sunshine. Lynne rents a small apartment within biking distance of her office. One day as she walks across campus, she's surprised by a sudden feeling of unease. She feels like she's stepping onto an unsteady boat. The sensation passes quickly. When she arrives at her office, she notices that some of the pictures are slightly tilted. She asks a nearby student whether she has just experienced her first earthquake. The student laughs and says, "Oh, that little sway was just a tremor, nothing like a *real* earthquake. Just wait until you're in a big one; it's totally awesome."

"Awesome? Are you kidding?" Lynne trembles, her heart races, and she begins to sweat. She hadn't considered the reality of earthquakes in California. She wonders if she can possibly cope. She recalls having used coping questions to deal with her anxiety about moving. Now she returns to these questions to help her calm her newly heightened fears about earthquakes.

Have I ever dealt with anything like this in the past?

No, I haven't. I don't think I can stand this. Maybe I need to quit and go back to dreary London.

How much will this affect my life a year from now?

Well, if I live through an earthquake, I guess I may be okay. If I don't, then I'll be dead.

Do I know people who've coped with something like this, and how did they do it?

I guess about 40 million or so Californians have lived through a few earthquakes and haven't moved out. They must have accepted the risk and learned to live with it.

Do I know anyone I could turn to for help or support?

I can ask people I know about earthquake safety and get more involved in the local neighborhood so I meet some of my neighbors.

Can I think of a creative new possibility that could result from this challenge?

I realize that lots of people come to the University of California from other countries around the world. Maybe I can start a group for new residents. We can socialize a bit and have speakers about adjusting to America, including earthquake safety. It will be a great way to meet new and interesting people and provide a way for me to expose myself to my fear.

Lynne learns to accept the risk of earthquakes and the questions help her to stop feeling helpless and anxious. See Chapter 6 for examples of how these questions can help you ponder and cope even with the possibility of an unexpected event that results in death.

Going right at your worries

Exposure — facing your fears gradually over time — is probably the most powerful approach to dealing with fear and anxiety. (Chapter 9 covers exposure in detail.) We suggest applying this technique to your fear of natural disasters. Don't worry — obviously, we're not going to recommend that you actually chase tornadoes or set forest fires and walk into them.

TIP

When dealing with a fear of natural disasters, the best exposure strategy is called *imaginal exposure*, which includes imagining the worst-case scenario (see Chapter 9). You can use imaginal exposure as an alternative approach to using the coping strategy questions (see the preceding section). Alejandro's story demonstrates how someone can apply imaginal exposure to an intense fear of earthquakes.

Alejandro lives in San Francisco. He worries about earthquakes. Rightly so, because San Francisco sits in a zone that poses a high risk for major earthquakes. Alejandro has taken all the usual, appropriate preparations, such as knowing how to shut off his utilities, securing water heater tanks, maintaining fire extinguishers, knowing evacuation routes, keeping emergency supplies, and such.

Nevertheless, he worries about earthquakes a lot. He jumps whenever he hears a rumble of thunder or an unexpected noise. His mind starts to dwell on horrible images of death and destruction, and then he quickly tries to think about something else.

Because he very much wants to continue living in San Francisco, Alejandro decides to see a psychologist. The psychologist suggests using imaginal exposure. At first, the strategy sounds to Alejandro like the psychologist is recommending that he do more of what's already scaring him — imagining scenes of horror and destruction. But the psychologist explains that imaginal exposure is different in a crucial manner. Imaginal exposure asks you to break your fears down into steps and gradually confront each one in your mind.

He tells Alejandro that he will hold the image of each step in his mind until his anxiety reduces somewhat. They start with the easiest step and work up from there. First, Alejandro and his psychologist spend part of the session talking about earthquakes. Just talking makes Alejandro nervous. Next, he finds a movie about earthquakes and watches it several times until he starts to get bored with it. By the next session, Alejandro is ready to imagine what it would feel like to experience an earthquake. He imagines a series of ever-worsening scenes of destruction and death, including his own demise. His psychologist facilitated the exposure by vividly describing details of an earthquake.

Note that some of Alejandro's steps occur solely in his imagination, and a few involve taking direct actions. By the time Alejandro has worked through multiple sessions of imaginal exposure, his anxiety about earthquakes decreases. He almost, really just *almost*, looks forward to coping with the next actual earthquake.

Doing Your Part to Improve the World

A number of research studies have shown that when people take charge of challenges and do something active, they cope better than if they cope passively. *Passive copers* usually do little more than try not to think about what worries them — this approach actually makes things worse for them.

On the other hand, *active copers* look for direct actions they can take to make themselves feel empowered. No, you can't actually do something to prevent most natural disasters like earthquakes, tsunamis, and volcanoes, but you can influence the environment for the better and/or improve the lives of other people who are threatened by disaster. Doing either of these things is likely to make you feel less like a helpless victim and more in charge of your concerns.

WARNING

If you decide to volunteer to either help the environment or victims of disasters (see the next two sections), you may encounter some difficulty or disappointment at first. Sometimes, volunteer organizations consist largely of people who've been with the organization a long time and who may not immediately welcome new members. It may take some time to win them over. In other cases, you may discover that your skills don't fit well with the group. Or you may find that your own shyness inhibits your efforts at first. So, we recommend that you give any such effort the time it takes to get over these concerns. You can also shop around until you find a comfortable fit.

Helping the environment

Maybe you're thinking that you, as one person, can't do much to affect the environment and natural disasters. But when millions of individuals each take steps to reduce the wear and tear on our planet, it adds up. So, taking action can help reduce your anxiety about natural disasters. You become part of the solution, not part of the problem.

First, consider all the ways you can decrease your own carbon footprint. Turn that thermostat down a little in the winter and up in the summer. Run your dishwasher only when it's totally full. Use electronic bill paying instead of paper. Eat less meat. Search the internet for a lot more ways to reduce your carbon footprint.

In addition, consider volunteering to help with the environment. Join a neighborhood trash-pickup effort. Volunteer for a conservation project. Help maintain a public walking trail. Get creative; you'll come up with other possibilities.

Volunteering in disasters

One way to feel more empowered is to become involved in planning for and providing service in the face of natural disasters. Your local Red Cross has many opportunities for volunteers. You can offer to answer phones, file papers, or provide direct assistance to people affected by disasters. The Red Cross offers training and education to help people gain the skills necessary to help others. Volunteering gives back. Helping others makes you feel more powerful and less anxious.

Chapter **16**

Racism and Anxiety

People have been oppressed since before the time of recorded history. Examples include slavery in biblical times, the oppression of serfs in feudal times, slavery in the New World, the internment of Japanese Americans during World War II, and the persecution of various indigenous people throughout human history. People have been oppressed on the basis of differences in race, gender, sexual identity, disability, ethnicity, geography, social class, or religion. This chapter mainly focuses on racial oppression, but the concepts can easily be applied to other ways of grouping people.

WARNING

We are two White authors. As such, we can't pretend to fully understand the experiences of people of color. Nor can we claim to be completely devoid of bias and racism. As much as we'd like to think of ourselves as anti-racists, because of our backgrounds, we understand the implicit bias that permeates even the best intended. Yet, we have hope. Recent protests represent continuations of the fight for equal rights that began decades ago. Clearly, far more needs to be done.

In this chapter, we describe the relationship between racism and anxiety. Racism can occur within institutions such as schools, police forces, political parties, governments, businesses, and professional sports. Racism can be expressed from one individual toward another. Victims of racism sometimes believe and even endorse racist messages through a process known as internalized racism.

We discuss how racism frequently leads to anxiety and other emotional problems. Interestingly, reported rates of anxiety are slightly lower among people of color. However, those rates are likely significantly underreported due to a lack of access to mental health care, culturally influenced perceived stigma for expressing mental health concerns, or fear of not being taken seriously by the healthcare system.

We provide tips for those who are targets of racism and dealing with the emotional toll. For those who want to help improve the world, we offer a couple ideas. We can only introduce you to a few key concepts about racism and anxiety in a single chapter. However, we urge you to pursue the topic in greater depth — today's world calls for increased attention and awareness of this critical issue. See the appendix for additional resources for rounding out your understanding of not only the role racism plays in anxiety, but also the way people relate to one another across the globe.

WARNING

We write about Black people, people of color, and White people almost as if they were all the same. Obviously, that's not the case as people have unique experiences and backgrounds that shape their attitudes and behaviors. Categorizing people into groups based on the color of their skin is fraught with danger. Our intent in using these global categories is to summarize typical experiences of group members, not to overly generalize or describe individual differences.

TECHNICAL STUFF

In ancient times, people were not categorized by physical differences. There is no genetic difference that clearly distinguishes one race from another. Race is primarily a socially defined concept.

Racism: The Elephant in the Room and the Snake in the Grass

Racism involves the erroneous belief that membership in specific racial or ethnic groups indicates inferiority or superiority in various abilities and attributes. The dominate group discriminates, exploits, antagonizes, and denies the oppressed group equal rights and access to power and privilege.

Racism can be blatant. Slur words, Confederate flags or monuments, Nazi symbols, hate-filled signs, burning crosses, and nooses are hard to misconstrue as anything but examples of racism. However, many people find thinking about or talking about racism excruciatingly uncomfortable. So, all too often, they ignore these messages, like an elephant in the room that everyone sees but pretends isn't there.

Other racist messages, like a snake in the grass, are stealthy and harder to detect. Examples of this sort of racism include failing to interview job applicants that have Black-sounding names or not calling back applicants of color after a positive interview. Real estate agents may not show Black buyers homes in certain neighborhoods. Other subtle biases include lower expectations coming from a racist belief that people of color may be less intelligent than their White counterparts. Racism emerges in various domains as seen in the following three sections.

REMEMBER

Both snakes and elephants create conditions of chronic stress and anxiety. The physical toll of this chronic stress can be seen in increased rates of various health problems experienced by people who are discriminated against.

Structural racism

Structural racism occurs across a range of tightly woven policies, norms, laws, institutions, governments, and beliefs that generate inequality and reduced opportunities for specific racial groups while privileging other groups. Just some of the examples of structural racism include:

>> Reduced educational opportunities due to unequal expenditures on schools located in diverse neighborhoods

>> Voter suppression through reduced access to polling places, excessively long lines — especially in diverse communities, purging of voter registration lists, and requiring picture identification to vote

>> Segregation whereby certain racial groups remain separate in schools and neighborhoods

>> Employment discrimination often resulting in lower wages and fewer prospects for career development and advancement

>> Lower wages, which flow directly from educational and employment inequities

>> Less wealth and savings, which leads to severe financial difficulty when emergencies occur or other unanticipated setbacks happen

>> Food deserts because major grocery stores are not located in poor neighborhoods, which leads to higher costs and lack of nutritious options contributing to poor health outcomes

>> Lack of adequate health insurance and healthcare

>> Even when insured, the insurance is often Medicaid, which provides more restricted access and benefits than private insurance or even Medicare

>> Reduced opportunities for homeownership and thus, reduced opportunity to accumulate wealth

>> U. S. immigration policies that favor White Europeans over immigrants of color

>> Tax policies that proportionally overtax low income families, especially through regressive sales taxes

>> The judicial system, which routinely imposes unrealistic bail, hands out longer sentences, and metes out harsher penalties to people of color

>> Police culture, which stops, frisks, arrests, targets, surveils, and with distressing frequency, assaults citizens of color more than White citizens

RACISM IN THE UK: THE WINDRUSH SCANDAL

The United Kingdom lost 384,00 soldiers and almost 70,000 civilians during World War II. London buildings were devastated by the German Blitz. With few able bodies to rebuild, the Brits called for immigrants from their colonies to help rebuild Great Britain. A group of Caribbean immigrants arrived in 1948 aboard the ship Windrush. They were builders, drivers, carpenters, maintenance workers, and nurses who provided much-needed help. They were also mostly Black.

More labor was needed in the early years of rebuilding. People from the colonies who arrived between 1948 and 1971 were called the Windrush Generation after the original ship. The Immigration Act of 1971 gave the Windrush generation permission to stay indefinitely. However, they were not given proper documentation of their status, and many old records were destroyed.

The Windrush scandal occurred as the British government became more conservative and restrictive with its immigration policies. Beginning in about 2013, it was reported that older Caribbean-born people were being asked for papers that they did not possess. Some were deported; others were detained. Members of the Windrush generation lost jobs, homes, and bank accounts while also being denied medical care. Their children, who grew up believing they were citizens (as promised to their parents), were asked for documentation proving that their parents had lived in the country prior to 1971. That was impossible for most, and the critics noted that they were "guilty until proven innocent."

Around 2017, newspapers began reporting on the scandal and some compensation has been paid to victims. However, critics maintain that much more needs to be done to address the plight of these people who had been recruited to help Great Britain recover. Many believe that structural racism was responsible for much of the undeserved maltreatment.

Factors such as these increase inequities and interact to produce more suffering. They create major impediments to persons of color who attempt to succeed and flourish. Structural racism envelopes people from birth until death, thus causing chronic stress, anxiety, and frustration.

WARNING

Again, it's important to realize that all individuals have different experiences. People of all races vary widely in terms of how and to what degree they experience or even perpetuate racism.

Interpersonal racism

Interpersonal racism is racism that occurs between individuals or small groups of people. It manifests itself in a variety of situations and settings. Studies have shown that interpersonal racism is a feature of everyday life for most people of color. Imagine living in a world in which few days go by without encountering some type of racist action or remark. There are two main types of interpersonal racism: overt and covert.

Overt racism

Overt interpersonal racism is obvious, blatant, unapologetic, discriminatory, hateful, and deliberate. Overt racism intends to intimidate those on the receiving end of it. It may involve threat, verbal abuse, symbols, ostracism, or physical aggression. These racist attitudes and ideas attempt to discriminate, humiliate, repudiate, and demean. Victims of overt racism, not surprisingly, suffer from anxiety, anger, disillusionment, fear, and hopelessness. Hate crimes are the most egregious form of overt racism. Hate crimes, which have been increasing over the last decade, involve offenses against people or property that is motivated by bias against particular races, religions, ethnicities, gender identity, or other perceived differences.

The Confederate flag is one example of overt racism, and is quite obviously so to most observers. However, some of those who display or carry the flag claim no racial intent at all. They claim the flag is a symbol of their heritage and nothing more. Whether they believe in their denial is an open question. Yet, the symbolic message of the flag to the descendants of former slaves is not at all unclear.

Covert racism

Unlike overt racism, covert racism is subtle and less blatantly obvious. When a security guard follows a Black teenager shopping at a mall, he may deny that he's following the teen because he's Black. However, deeply engrained prejudice likely contributes to his tendency to surveil certain shoppers more than others. Covert racism may involve unconsciously held stereotypes and attitudes about racial differences, such as subtle assumptions of criminality or inferiority.

A particularly impactful arena for covert racism occurs in the healthcare system. Black people have shorter lifespans and suffer more health problems than their White counterparts in the United States. Despite healthcare providers who deny racial bias, numerous studies have concluded that Black patients receive fewer interventions (such as radiation, coronary bypass operations, kidney dialysis, and so on), earlier discharges, and more conservative as opposed to cutting edge treatments. These disparities occur even when controlling for the influences of private health insurance, income, age, and severity of illness.

A FAMILY PHYSICIAN'S TAKE ON STRESS AND RACISM

We had a couple of discussions with LaTasha Seliby Perkins, M.D., a family physician and an assistant professor in the Department of Family Medicine at Georgetown University School of Medicine. Dr. Perkins has a keen interest in the toll that racism inflicts on the emotional and physical health of her Black patients. She stated that stress increases cortisol (the body's stress hormone), which can lead to high blood pressure, inflammation, and mental malaise. Dr. Perkins emphasized that Black patients need to open up and speak to their family physicians about their experiences of stress and racism. Family physicians can offer guidance and resources to their patients concerning these issues.

She had four specific recommendations for her Black patients experiencing stress and racism:

- Engage in physical exercise that includes 15–20 minutes of stretching to aid in the reduction of the negative effects of stress hormones.

- Practice mindfulness in a way that feels comfortable to you, such as mediation, breathing exercises, yoga, affirmations, or prayer.

- Consider social interactions or fellowship where you can share, grow, and heal in a communal environment versus isolation.

- If daily activities are significantly impacted by stress or anxiety, consider seeking the additional help of a mental health professional.

Dr. Perkins also emphasized the importance of parents' vigilance to their teens' moods, emotions, and behaviors. If they see problems with sleep, excessive worry, lack of interest in things that were once enjoyable, dropping grades, isolation, or acting out, it may suggest the need for a discussion with their family physician or a mental health professional. Finally, she suggested that teens of color could benefit from a trustworthy, culturally aware confidant.

TECHNICAL STUFF

Microaggression is a term that's frequently used to describe a type of covert racism. Microaggressions have been defined as common, everyday insults or affronts, sometimes intentional but sometimes not, directed toward marginalized individuals or groups.

Internalized racism

When someone has been exposed to racism over a lifetime, it comes as no surprise that racist beliefs sometimes become incorporated into the recipient's own self-image. Repeated messages of denigration may lead to feelings of self-doubt, inferiority, or undesirability. A tragic form of internalized racism occurs when people of color are convinced that they cannot achieve because they lack ability. This leads to feelings of helplessness and may decrease ambition. Another example of internalized racism includes attempts to appear "whiter" with skin lightening products or hair straightening. (See the sidebar "Colorism" for more information.)

Other examples can be found in people of color who endorse racial stereotypes such as believing that all Blacks possess athletic ability or that Black people are somehow less intelligent than White people. Internalized racism is associated with high levels of psychological distress and anxiety.

COLORISM

Racism is not just a problem in the United States. Throughout India, South Asia, and Africa, many women use cosmetics to lighten their skin. Lighter skin tones have been associated with an ideal of beauty that has been encouraged by the billion-dollar skin "whitening or lightening" industry. Some major cosmetics companies have bowed to recent social pressures and have changed the names and marketing of such products. However, they as yet have not taken the more meaningful step of discontinuing their manufacture.

Women with dark skin have reported being ostracized and traumatized because of the social bias associated with their skin color. The formidable and ubiquitous influence of this bias even shows up in some internet dating sites that have allowed prospective dates to be filtered according to skin tone. One such site shut down this filter following the killing of George Floyd and subsequent protests. In India, Bollywood (the nickname of India's film industry) has shown a preference for light-skinned stars. This predilection supports the bias against dark-skinned beauty.

How Racism Leads to Anxiety

Chronic stress leads to anxiety. Daily experiences of racism cause stress. These experiences are continuous, chronic, and cumulative. People of color are often subject to racism while living their normal routine lives. Some of the more well-known instances of public racism happen in the following situations:

» **Driving while Black:** African-American men experience a higher rate of being pulled over by police for minor traffic infractions such as a rolling stop, a broken taillight, or an expired license plate than White Americans. Many are also stopped for suspicious behavior (such as driving a nice car in a nice neighborhood). These reports are substantiated by police statistics. Unfortunately, these minor infractions sometimes have resulted in violence, arrests, and occasionally death.

» **Sleeping while Black:** A college graduate student took a nap after studying in her dorm common room. Upon seeing her asleep, a classmate woke her up and told her that she shouldn't be there. She then called campus police. An incident in Atlanta, Georgia, involved a Black man sleeping in his car. This minor incident escalated into a violent confrontation in which the man was shot in the back and killed as he attempted to run away.

» **Walking while Black:** New York City used to routinely stop and frisk Black and Brown citizens who were committing the crime of walking on the sidewalk. Although the official policy has been discontinued, many people of color report being stopped for suspicious activity, frisked, and questioned, sometimes followed by arrest or even a violent confrontation.

» **Drinking coffee while Black:** Two Black men entered a coffee shop to pass time before a business meeting. They were asked to leave and refused to do so. Police were called who came and surrounded the men. They were arrested on the charge of suspicion of trespassing. The coffee shop company apologized and declined to have the men charged.

» **Birdwatching while Black:** A Black man bird watching in Central Park asked a White woman to put a leash on her dog (which is the law in New York City). She responded by calling 911 and telling them that an African-American man was threatening her and her dog. It was determined that his behavior was appropriate because he had recorded the entire incident on his phone. However, this incident reflects the daily stress that people of color face.

» **Police encounters while Black:** Government statistics show that African-American men and women, Native American men and women, and Latino men all face a higher lifetime risk of being killed by police officers than White men or women or Latina women. African-American men are at the highest risk of police violence. Minneapolis has a population of about 430,000. Twenty percent of people in Minneapolis are African American. However, 60 percent of the physical violence of police toward citizens targets African Americans.

These are but a few of a long series of well-known incidents that occur frequently in the lives of people of color. Countless, everyday harassments and biased treatment accumulate and fuel a sense of being under attack and a need to be constantly vigilant for the next incident. This hypervigilance leads to burdensome levels of stress and anxiety that those in the dominate culture often fail to perceive or understand.

However, many people of color do not seek help for their anxiety. People of color often prefer to deal with their emotional issues on their own or by seeking help from family, friends, or spiritual leaders. That may have to do with the stigma of admitting to emotional problems.

It's also speculated that avoidance of care may stem from a lack of trust in the healthcare system and a paucity of qualified therapists of similar ethnic background. In addition, lack of financial resources or health insurance further constrains utilization of mental health resources. Other barriers to seeking treatment for mental health issues include lack of paid sick time, problems getting childcare, reduced mental health services in many minority areas, and lack of reliable transportation.

Not seeking help for anxiety may also lead to an exacerbation of underlying physical problems. People with chronic, untreated anxiety report higher blood pressure, elevated heart rate, difficulty concentrating, tension headaches, muscle tension, stomach upsets, fatigue, insomnia, and problems with appetite. In addition, whether due to stress, genetics, experienced racism, or other causes, people of color experience a greater range of health disparities that lead to more chronic illnesses and in many cases a shorter life span.

TIP

When we talk about anxiety, especially the anxiety of those who are subject to racism, we prefer not to use the term "anxiety disorder." That's because anxiety seems to be a perfectly rational reaction to constant stress and menace caused by racism. That same principle applies to much of mental illness that is a product of individuals as they interact with a challenging world.

RACISM AGAINST FIRST PEOPLES

Early explorers to the New World brought death, disease, and starvation to the indigenous of the area. Explorers were given permission to conquer indigenous people by a Papal declaration that promoted the conquest, colonization, and mass conversion of all non-Christians throughout the world. It is estimated that before European settlers invaded, at least ten to twelve million indigenous people thrived in North America. By the time the Europeans claimed North America as their own, they had displaced and massacred millions. *By the 1890s, the indigenous population had plummeted to about 300,000.*

These genocides have been and are disturbingly common throughout the world as one group conquers another. Land and natural resources are stolen and never returned. Some native groups have been able to negotiate partial reparations, but rarely does the compensation amount to more than a token sum.

Consider the original people from the island of Manhattan. They gave up their lands and moved to Pennsylvania. Later they moved west to Ohio, then west to Indiana, finally settling in Kansas. When the American government decided that land in Kansas was too valuable, they moved to a rural area of Oklahoma. This is a typical pattern of forcing indigenous people to move from precious land to land with little value. We're guessing they weren't well compensated for their New York City real estate.

Coping with Racism

Racism and discrimination are ubiquitous in the United States and around the world. Racism should not exist. And it is unfair that those who suffer from racism are asked to cope with it. We believe that for real change, racism must be fought in the institutions that perpetuate it and among the individuals, communities, and nations that support racism. However, until these changes are successful, targets of racism must find ways to cope.

Although the targets of racism may differ, the impact on victims is profound. People who experience racism feel isolated, intimidated, anxious, angry, and enraged. Although the burden of change should lie with the oppressors, the oppressed usually shoulder most of the responsibility for their own, individual coping. They are also left with too much of the burden of changing society at large and encouraging others to become true allies of change. Nevertheless, engaged, empowered coping with racism is likely to decrease frustration and improve mental health overall.

Finding empowerment

Empowerment means living with the expectation that all people are created equal and *should* have certain rights. Empowered people have pride in their cultural group and seek knowledge about their own racial/ethnic experience. They identify with their race as well as their other roles in the culture. They think of themselves as complex individuals with multiple perspectives. In other words, all people are not simply members of a single group (racial, ethnic, religious, and so forth); they're also mothers, fathers, sons, daughters, and workers. Thus, they have multiple identities and viewpoints.

Empowered people of color understand the impact of racism and stand up to challenge the inequities. They actively engage with individuals, institutions, and the culture to assert their right to equality. Empowerment is the antithesis of feeling victimized. Empowerment can be enhanced by engagement, increased political participation, protesting, and joining activist groups.

WARNING

People of color have many positive reasons to engage in mass protests. The exact risks of protesting during a pandemic are unclear. However, health risks are known to be higher for Black and Brown people. People have to choose their own tolerance for risk in making the decision to protest.

Empowerment can occur on an individual level by standing up to an offensive statement or offering divergent opinions. An empowered person may choose to leave a situation or group in which discrimination occurs, and repeated demands for change go unheeded.

Self-education is an important part of empowerment. Empowered people seek knowledge about activist groups as well as the political process. Organizing and seeking like-minded people increases the sense of empowerment for all concerned.

Persistence forms the foundation of empowerment. No matter how critical the issue, altering systems requires extraordinary, sustained effort to bring about meaningful change. And numerous setbacks are the norm. For example, the South African struggle against Apartheid took more than 40 years, and much remains to be done even after the formal segregated system fell in the early 1990s.

Staying connected

The effects of racism on those who experience it include anxiety, pessimism, and depression. Friends, family, mentors, or others who share similar experiences can offer social support, which improves coping. Copers surround themselves with people who value them and know their worth. Whether the support involves discussion around the kitchen table, over coffee with friends, or in a political discussion group designed to discuss racism, expressing feelings and thoughts with others often facilitates healing.

In addition to talking about racism, many people want to do something directly to express their frustration and work for change. Protests have been a catalyst for change throughout history. The aspect of doing something with a large group of people provides a feeling of empowerment as well as camaraderie. Getting involved in a political campaign or social action group also provides meaningful interactions with others as well as a sense of purpose.

Almost 80 percent of African Americans identify themselves as Christian. The church supports the idea of equality and peace among all people. Many Black Christians find solace in the church's message. Church gatherings or spiritual counseling offer a source of critical social support for those who experience the frustration, grief, and sadness of discrimination. Black churches often provide unique opportunities for open emotional expression and connections for their congregations.

Accepting emotion

Research on emotional suppression has typically demonstrated that suppression leads to greater health impairments such as high blood pressure, reduced immunity, and higher risk for cardiovascular events. Furthermore, avoidance of emotion tends to be a temporary fix. After the initial suppression, the emotion is likely to come roaring back.

A few decades ago, a popular treatment for anger targeted the idea of emotional expression as being important for mental health. Lots of people yelled into pillows, threw items in a padded room, or screamed as loud as they could. Primal scream therapy, as it was known as, did not appear to work. In fact, expressing anger in that way actually increases unfocused anger. So, why the contradiction? Do you express your emotions or inhibit them?

The answer lies in whether your anger can be expressed in a productive manner, with a goal or purpose. Screaming your rage into a pillow doesn't do much for understanding or changing the original cause. However, marching in protest, boycotting, or expressing yourself can do much to put your anger to use.

REMEMBER

Other emotions such as anxiety, depression, and grief also need to be acknowledged, expressed, and accepted. See Chapter 8 for information about accepting and tolerating emotions.

Taking care of yourself

Social support, becoming empowered, and accepting emotions are three ways to deal with racism. However, sometimes the stress of being the target of discrimination and bias becomes overwhelming. It's normal to feel sad or angry as a result of the painful experiences of racism. People who do better emotionally accept their feelings because they're appropriate.

There are healthy ways to cope. On the other hand, it could be tempting to check out and avoid pain by consuming drugs or alcohol — or becoming isolated and withdrawn. But in the long run, those escapes do little to deal with the underlying feelings. Finding activities that increase strength, resilience, and serenity works best. For some, finding strength, resilience, and serenity means a spiritual practice, for others it involves charity, and still others find peace in jogging. Others find solace by practicing forgiveness when it frees them and give thanks for what they do have.

TIP

If, in spite of your best efforts, you find yourself overwhelmed by emotions (as appropriate as they may be), it may be useful to consult with a mental health professional. This is especially true if your emotions are interfering with everyday functioning at home or work. Ideally, consider seeking a professional who has training in multicultural issues. If available, you may want to seek a therapist that shares your background.

Fighting Racism

Silence about racism is accepting racism. Dealing with racism is powerfully uncomfortable, but silence indirectly supports it. Far too many people in the majority culture believe they can safely ignore discrimination, bias, and blatant racism and consider themselves as non-racist because they don't personally engage in such actions. In their minds, they are, in effect, comfortably "color blind." However, not acknowledging that unfairness, discrimination, and exploitation leads to societal and institutional support of the status quo. And the status quo is racially toxic for a large percentage of our fellow citizens.

Becoming an ally

Many White people feel that because they don't consciously endorse racist ideas they are allies of people of color. In order to become an ally, White people should consider understanding their privileged status. What that means is that White people have inherent advantages. These advantages include, for the most part, better schools, more stable neighborhoods, fair treatment by police, and the absence of frequent discrimination.

The first step of becoming an ally is to understand that even if you didn't directly participate in the creation of historical racism, you can still take action. You can speak against the inherent unfairness that's been imposed on your fellow citizens for centuries.

Besides, there are advantages to those who advocate for transforming racial relations. To begin with, inclusiveness provides for a wider range of perspectives, which can facilitate problem-solving and increase creativity. Furthermore, a more equitable society will likely increase stability, improve individual adjustment, decrease social unrest, and increase productivity. The bottom line: Improved racial justice will no doubt create a better world for all of us.

Educating yourself

In order to fight racism, it is important to become educated about the historical and current experiences of people of color. Through reading, watching documentaries, engaging, and reflecting on racism you can begin to understand racism more deeply. (See the appendix for resources about racism.)

You may even discover that you possess beliefs that appear racist even though your intentions are not racist. Open your mind to the possibility that your own actions or inactions may have contributed to oppression. We say this not to engender guilt and shame, but rather to push us all toward a more fair and equitable society. What matters is not where you started, but where you end up. We can all do better.

Speaking up

Speaking up against racism requires courage. Mistakes are inevitable. Decide what you want to communicate and mentally practice doing so. Don't attack the person, but comment on what you find offensive. You can't expect instant agreement and may even get counterattacked. Realize that change is hard and takes time. You will not get instant gratification very often.

Set limits on what you're willing to accept. For example, it's perfectly alright to tell family or friends that you do not want to hear racist jokes or comments in your presence. You may give a reminder or two, and you also may ultimately have to leave the person or situation you're in.

When possible, speak to the person's values. For example, if someone categorizes a group of people in a derogatory manner (such as lazy), you might say, "You usually try to be fair minded, so I'm confused why you're labeling a whole ethnic group as lazy. I find that offensive and would rather not hear it."

At the same time, it's often useless to argue with a person who makes blatantly racist statements. Arguments typically end up with both sides defensive and stuck. It's better to state your opinion, be direct and label the behavior as offensive, set appropriate limits, and move on.

Sometimes people who are attempting to be anti-racist may say something that is inadvertently racist. It may be a phrase from childhood or an inadvertent slip. If you say something offensive, own up and apologize. Avoid defensiveness. Learn from your mistake and strive to do better.

Teaching your children well

Talk to your kids about race from early on. Make the effort to purchase children's books with a diversity of characters. Because of still existing segregation, many young children have had little or no exposure to people of different races or ethnicities. Consider sending young children to day care and schools that have a diverse population.

Talk to your children about issues such as fairness, equality, and inclusion. When discrimination is encountered, whether through media or in person, take the time to discuss the implications with your children. Ask questions about how those who are mistreated may feel. Even young children grasp the concept of fairness.

Exploring the unfamiliar

Don't limit your exposure to diverse people by simply going to ethnic festivals or restaurants (although by all means, go to them, have fun, and enjoy)! But exposure means much more. Try to frequent businesses that are owned by people of color. Travel to places where you will obviously stand out as a minority. Consider joining a club or interest group that has diverse membership. Take classes on topics such as Minority Politics, Urban History, History of Slavery, or African-American Literature. Expand your horizons.

REMEMBER

The stress from racism impacts everyone. Whether you encounter direct discrimination or observe its affect on others, racism degrades the emotional and physical health of society at large.

Chapter **17**

Keeping Out of Danger

U nexpected events frighten most people from time to time. Have you ever been in an airplane when turbulence caused a sudden dip of the plane as well as your stomach? Or watched in slow motion as another car careened across the road sliding in your direction? How about noticing someone wearing dark clothing, who's nervously glancing around, sweating, and carrying a large bag at a ticket counter? Do you get a bit jumpy in a strange city in the dark, not sure which way to go? On a crowded subway, when someone starts coughing and sneezing, do you feel queasy, tense, and suddenly want to jump off at the next stop?

This chapter is about anxiety related to dangers via violence, accidents, crime, and diseases and the emotional aftermath of fearing the worst. First, we take a look at your personal risks — just how safe you are and how you can improve your odds. Then we discuss methods you can use to prepare or help yourself in the event that something traumatic happens to you. Finally, we talk about acceptance, a path to calmness and serenity in the face of an uncertain world.

Evaluating Your Actual, Personal Risks

The risk of experiencing natural disasters is quite low for most people. But lots of people worry about them nonetheless. Interestingly, the same can be said about risks of terrorism. Billions of dollars are spent each year trying to combat terrorism. Billions of dollars are also spent every year on crime prevention. And more people worry about getting hurt or dying as the result of crime, natural disasters, or terrorism than the real leading causes of death. The actual leading causes of death include

>> Cardiovascular disease (about 32 percent of all causes of death)

>> Cancer (about 20 percent)

>> Respiratory diseases and infections (about 12 percent with the exception of pandemics)

In fact, disease is responsible for about 85 percent of all deaths. By contrast, terrorism, violent crime, and natural disasters account for less than 1 percent of all deaths worldwide in a typical year. So, why do people worry so much more about these violent ways of dying than the actual common causes of death? The answer lies deep within the human brain. The brain processes an overwhelming amount of information. In order to handle that data efficiently, it attempts to sort information by priorities. The brain's primary priority is to avoid danger and pain.

Therefore, any information related to those issues is highlighted and processed quickly and efficiently. Dramatic events (such as terrorist attacks, violent crime, or natural disasters) are more attention-grabbing than the long, slow disease processes that more typically lead to death. See Chapter 13 for information about cognitive biases that greatly impede the ability to accurately sort through information.

Bottom line, your own risk of death depends on a variety of factors, including

>> **Genetics:** Some families pass down genes that are related to high rates of cancer, diabetes, heart disease, or other less common health conditions. If you carry such genetic risks, you can often make adjustments to your lifestyle to mitigate them.

>> **Lifestyle:** This includes your diet, exercise, stress management, career choice, and quality of your relationships.

>> **Environment and cultural influences:** This component includes air and water quality, risks for natural disasters, climate, educational opportunities, crime, political conditions, and discrimination or racism.

Avoiding Unnecessary Risks

Accidents happen, and people get sick. And eventually, as far as we know, everyone dies. Whatever your own personal beliefs are about what happens after death, most people don't look forward to dying. Some believe that people have a certain amount of time on this planet and what they do with their day-to-day lives doesn't much matter.

But how you live your life greatly affects your health and comfort, no matter what happens in the end, whereas worry never kept anyone healthy. So, we recommend that you take a careful look at your lifestyle, take whatever steps you can to minimize those risks, and then make the best you can out of each and every day.

REMEMBER

So far, no one has been able to predict the future. Live each day fully and to the best of your ability. Worry and regret do not lead to better health.

Actions for keeping health risks low

Decide what steps you can take to improve your chances of having a long, healthy life. Don't try and tackle everything at once. The following examples can guide you:

>> If you're inactive, don't plan on running the next marathon; start by walking 15 minutes a day, most days a week.

>> If you have a family history of high cholesterol, get a referral to a dietician to talk about ways to improve your diet.

>> Buy sunscreen and wear it every day. Daily use of sunscreen has the added benefit of keeping your skin looking young.

>> Floss your teeth; it does more for your health than you think!

>> Keep on trying to quit smoking. It may take lots of effort, but millions of people eventually do quit; you can too.

>> Add one more serving of fruits and vegetables to your diet.

>> Don't put off medical screening tests — especially mammograms and colonoscopies.

>> Follow public health guidelines, especially during a global health crisis.

>> If you do get sick, be hopeful and optimistic.

>> Stay connected with friends and family.

>> Accept the fact that life and death are part of this world.

Actions for keeping daily life risks low

No matter what your risks for experiencing violence, we advise taking reasonable precautions to keep yourself safe. A little preparation usually doesn't cost a lot in terms of either time or money. The key is making active decisions about what seems reasonable and then trying to let your worry go because you've done what makes sense. If, instead, you listen to the anxious, obsessional part of your mind, you'll never stop spending time preparing — and needlessly upset your life in the process.

We suggest the following, fully realizing that some of these may sound a little obvious. But because people often don't follow these suggestions, here they are:

>> Wear seat belts; need we say more?

>> If you have a wallet, carry it in your front pocket. Hold onto purses and bags.

>> If you're traveling, research the area for known risks. The U.S. State Department lists areas deemed unsafe for travel because of terrorism or other known risks at http://travel.state.gov.

>> Drive safely, and adhere to all traffic rules. Don't drive if fatigued or impaired in any other way.

>> Make copies of your passport; give one to someone before you leave and put another in your luggage separate from the bag you carry.

>> Don't wear expensive jewelry when you travel.

>> Don't drive in terrible weather conditions.

>> Consider carrying a loud whistle in your purse or pocket.

>> Heed the oft-given advice to report any unattended baggage in airports, train stations, or hotel lobbies.

>> Be careful of public Wi-Fi; don't enter sensitive, financial, or personal information. Be careful about posting vacation activities on social media until you arrive at home.

>> If you're in a hotel room, don't answer the door unless you know who it is. If you're not sure, call the front desk.

>> If you do have to walk in an unsafe area, walk quickly and pay attention.

>> Have your keys out and ready as you approach your car, and look before you get in.

>> Try not to walk alone in dark, secluded areas.

REMEMBER

Don't limit your ability to enjoy life. Realize some risks are inevitable. Consider travel to places other than your backyard! Get to know some people from other cultures and lands. See some interesting landscapes. In other words, don't wall yourself off from the world.

Dealing with Trauma-Related Anxiety

We hope you're never a victim of nor a witness to severe violence, but we know it's a real possibility. Violence occurs in war, on the streets, and even in the work-place. So if you've recently been a victim, you may be experiencing some serious signs of anxiety or distress. That reaction is pretty normal. And the first thing we're going to tell you is that, *unless your symptoms are quite severe* and interfering greatly with your life, don't seek out mental health treatment right away! That's because, in many cases, your mind's own natural healing process will suffice.

WARNING

Furthermore, it's quite easy to interfere with natural recovery. For example, a single *debriefing session* often takes place after exposure to a traumatic event. In such a session, people are given basic information about trauma and its potential effects and are then encouraged to talk about how they're coping with it. But such a session may actually increase the risk of emotional symptoms occurring or con-tinuing. If you're offered such a single-session intervention, we suggest skipping it unless it's obligatory. It's perfectly okay not to want to talk about the trauma right away.

So here's what we recommend you do first if you're unfortunate enough to wit-ness or experience a highly traumatic event:

>> Realize that it's normal to feel fearful and distressed.

>> Talk to people you feel comfortable discussing the trauma with, but don't let yourself be pressured to talk by anyone.

>> Ask yourself what you've done in the past to get through tough times and see whether that helps you get through this one. For example, some people find benefit from spiritual counseling, prayer, turning to friends, or increasing exercise.

>> If you're experiencing severe symptoms such as flashbacks, serious insom-nia, significant irritability, or anxiety after a few months (even sooner if the symptoms are highly disturbing), consider seeing a mental health profes-sional. Be sure to ask whether your therapist uses *evidence-based* treatment. Evidence-based treatment refers to therapies that have been supported by empirical, scientific research.

WARNING

The following sections discuss strategies for dealing with anxiety that results from exposure to some type of trauma. Sometimes this anxiety evolves into a more serious condition called post-traumatic stress disorder (PTSD). PTSD requires professional intervention. So, if your anxiety is particularly intense and/or seriously interferes with your life functioning, seek a professional diagnosis and treatment.

Thinking through what happened

When people have been exposed to trauma, the experience sometimes lingers. But with time and effort, the anxiety can decrease, and life satisfaction gets much better.

Take a hard look back and think about the meaning that the traumatic event had for you in your life. In other words, describe how you think your life has changed for the worse or for the better:

>> Do you feel responsible for the trauma?

>> Do you feel unsafe everywhere you go?

>> Have you managed to acquire a new value and/or purpose in your life?

>> Have you changed the way you feel about yourself as a person?

>> Are you angry, sad, or ashamed?

Explore your feelings and how your thoughts may be contributing to making things worse than they need to be for you. Among other things, ask these questions:

>> How does this event affect the way you see yourself and the world?

>> What would you tell a friend that this event meant about him or her as a person? Can you accept saying the same thing to yourself?

>> Do you know anyone who has coped with something like this? If so, how did they do it?

>> Do you believe that you're more unsafe than anyone else? If so, what is the evidence that you are?

>> Did you *want* this traumatic event to happen to you? If not, can you stop blaming yourself?

>> Is there anything shameful about having been a victim of trauma or violence?

>> Can you think of a creative new possibility that could result from this challenge? For example, could you volunteer to help others in similar situations?

Exposing yourself to the incident

Exposure therapy, as we describe in Chapter 9, has been supported by more research studies than any other approach for treating anxiety. Briefly, *exposure therapy* involves making extended contact with the feared or traumatic event, sometimes through imagery.

The main problem with this approach lies in the fact that lots of trauma victims really don't want to revisit their trauma. Thus, the very idea of exposure elicits feelings of great distress. For some, exposure seems like adding more suffering to their already traumatized lives. For that reason, among others, far too many trauma victims fail to get treatment.

TIP

If you find that the prospect of exposure therapy seems completely overwhelming to you, consider seeking professional help.

Accepting a Certain Degree of Uncertainty

Emotional distress stemming from traumas, whether from accidents, health crises, or violence, presents a challenge, yet it's quite normal. It's important to realize that people can't control the emotions that arise from such causes. The more you can accept that fact, the more easily you'll be able to cope with life and whatever it deals you. The next two sections take a look at accepting uncertainty and risk.

Choosing to put yourself in high-risk situations

Some people, like police officers, emergency medical personnel, soldiers, and firefighters, choose to expose themselves to the best and worst of life. Their motives are positive. They may have a strong desire to help others, feel a deep sense of patriotism, or want to make a positive difference in the world. These people often become anxious or even traumatized by the horrible events and disasters that they must deal with.

Those who fully understand and accept both the risks of the job and the fact that they may experience emotional distress from exposure to trauma just may be a little less vulnerable to traumatic events than those who see themselves as invincible. Paradoxically, the more you can accept whatever responses you have, the more easily you'll deal with them.

However, those who view themselves as indestructible may actually choose to go into their fields with an inflated sense of invulnerability. These people are more likely to have emotional pain from their experiences and refuse or shun help. They believe that part of their job is to handle whatever happens to them. Sadly, they're not immune to horror and trauma, yet they think that they should be.

REMEMBER

If you or someone you care about has a front-line position in a field like medical care, law enforcement, or the military, you're at risk, just like everyone else, for getting a stress disorder from exposure to horrible events. This doesn't make you weak or less competent. You must bravely face your emotional pain and get help. Denying the emotional pain dulls your ability to continue to help others.

Experiencing danger in everyday places

A lot of people live lives in which they try to stay away from danger. But life happens to them as well. People are exposed to violence in places that were once considered safe: schools, churches, synagogues, mosques, parks, and the work-place. In addition, unexpected health threats, accidents, and natural disasters are a part of life. *Uncertainty in this world is certain.*

The only alternative to acceptance of risk and uncertainty is to devote your entire life to anticipating and avoiding risk. The problem here is that your efforts will still fail. Even if you spend every waking moment trying to avoid risk, it won't work. So far, we know of no one who has managed to avoid the ultimate risk of death.

The following story illustrates typical symptoms of stress and anxiety following a motor vehicle accident.

> **Lew** had always assumed, like most people do, that a green light signals it's safe to proceed through an intersection. He had driven with that assumption for 20 years without mishap. One day on the way to work, Lew drives through an intersection that he has safely traversed hundreds of times before. Suddenly, an SUV barrels through the red light and broadsides Lew's sedan. Lew suffers serious injuries. After several weeks in the hospital, he spends months in rehabilitation.
>
> When Lew returns to driving, he finds himself creeping through intersections with intense feelings of anxiety. He can barely make himself drive to work and back each day and avoids driving whenever possible. His body aches with tension. He's irritable and moody.

UNUSUAL, UNPREDICTABLE ENDINGS

Consider asking yourself how you could avoid these calamitous yet impossible-to-predict events. Please realize that we're not trying to be funny about or make light of tragic, violent, and horrific events. Our point is simply that you can never know how to predict and avoid the unpredictable. As we said, life has risks.

- A vacationing couple was left in the Great Barrier Reef off the coast of Australia when a dive boat crew member failed to count them upon returning to the boat — their bodies were never recovered.

- A surgeon in Houston was decapitated by an elevator door closing on his head.

- A 28-year-old woman died of drinking too much water in a radio station contest.

- An employee fell into a large tank of hot, melting chocolate and died after being knocked unconscious by one of the mixing paddles.

- A chef in China died after a bite from a cobra's head. He had just beheaded the snake in order to make soup.

- A lawyer threw himself into a glass window to prove that the glass was unbreakable; unfortunately, he discovered that the windowpanes themselves broke out, and he fell from the 24th floor of the building.

- Every player on a soccer team in Africa was killed instantly by a forked bolt of lightning.

- A 24-year-old was trying to heat up a lava lamp on his kitchen stove; it exploded with such force that a shard of glass pierced his heart and killed him.

- Nine people were killed when over a million liters of beer burst out of a huge vat, causing a chain reaction that ripped open surrounding vats of beer and flooded the streets. The flood of beer filled surrounding houses and pubs, drowning those in its path. The BBC referred to the event as a beer tsunami; it's more commonly known as the London Beer Flood of 1814.

- And if you think the London Beer Flood sounds bad, there's always the Boston Molasses Tragedy. In 1919, 2.3 million gallons of molasses burst through a large storage tank and resulted in a wall of molasses about 15 to 20 feet high, wiping out homes and buildings and trapping people in the sweet goo. Twenty people were killed and about 150 injured. Months later, globs of molasses still clung to doors, sidewalks, and streets.

Lew's doctor tells him that he now has high blood pressure and that he needs to reduce his stress. Lew worries about his worry but doesn't know what he can do about it. He thinks he may have to take a leave of absence from work. His supervisor is losing patience with him. Desperate, Lew makes another appointment with his doctor. This time, the doctor takes time to ask Lew about his symptoms. He refers Lew to a psychotherapist who specializes in working with people with anxiety and trauma for an evaluation and treatment.

The therapist recommends exposure therapy (see the earlier section "Exposing yourself to the incident") involving a series of steps that start with talking about the accident and gradually increase in difficulty up to repeatedly driving through busy intersections.

The therapist then works on helping Lew develop *acceptance.* He works with Lew to see that feelings are just feelings, not something to be avoided. He teaches Lew how to remain in contact with his emotions without judging them. Lew gradually learns to accept his emotions for what they are. The more Lew accepts his anxiety, the less it bothers him. He now can drive with reasonable comfort through almost any intersection.

5

Helping Others with Anxiety

Recognize anxiety in friends and family.

Assist without taking over.

Recognize normal anxiety versus a problem.

Reduce the risk of anxiety exploding.

Know when to get help for kids.

IN THIS CHAPTER

» **Finding out whether your partner or a friend has anxiety**

» **Communicating about anxiety**

» **Coaching your anxious acquaintance**

» **Working together to fight anxiety**

» **Accepting your anxious friend or family member**

Chapter **18**

When a Family Member or Friend Suffers from Anxiety

Perhaps your friend, partner, or relative gets irritated easily, avoids going out with you, or often seems distant and preoccupied. Possibly he seems overly worried about sickness, money, or safety. Maybe he shuns physical intimacy. Or he may leave parties, concerts, or sports events early for no apparent reason.

You could easily take his behavior personally. You may think he doesn't love you, care about you, or is angry with you. And if these behaviors represent a recent change, it's difficult to know what's going on for sure. But it could be that your friend or partner actually suffers from anxiety.

This chapter helps you figure out whether someone you care about suffers from anxiety. We also help you communicate effectively with a loved one who has anxiety. With the right communication style, instead of provoking feelings of anger and resentment, you may be able to negotiate a new role — that of a helpful coach. You can also team up to tackle anxiety by finding ways to simplify life, have fun, and relax together. Finally, we explain how simply accepting your partner's anxiety and limitations leads to a better relationship and, surprisingly, less anxiety.

TIP

For convenience and clarity in this chapter, we mostly use the term "loved one" to refer to any partner, friend, or relative that you may be concerned about.

When Your Loved One Suffers from Anxiety

People who live together sometimes don't know each other as well as they think they do. Most people try to look and act as well adjusted as they can, because revealing weaknesses, limitations, and vulnerabilities isn't easy. Why do people hide their anxious feelings? Two big reasons for hiding them include

>> **Fear:** Revealing negative feelings can be embarrassing, especially to someone with an anxiety disorder. People often fear rejection or ridicule, even though self-disclosure usually brings people closer together.

>> **Upbringing:** Children may have been taught to repress or deny feelings by their parents. They may have been told, "Don't be such a baby," or "Boys don't cry." When taught to hide feelings, people grow up keeping concerns to themselves.

So, how do you really know whether your loved one has a problem with anxiety? And does it matter whether you know or not? We think it does. Understanding whether your partner experiences anxiety promotes better communication and facilitates closeness.

The following list of indications may help you to discern whether your partner suffers from anxiety. Ask yourself whether your partner

>> Seems restless and keyed up

>> Avoids situations for seemingly silly reasons

>> Ruminates about future catastrophes

>> Is reluctant to leave the house

>> Has trouble sleeping or staying asleep

>> Has trouble concentrating

>> Is plagued with self-doubts

>> Has episodes of noticeable shakiness and distress

- >> Is constantly on alert for dangers

- >> Seems unusually touchy about criticism

- >> Is overly worried about getting sick

- >> Seems unusually concerned about health

- >> Has frequent, unexplained bouts of nausea, dizziness, or aches and pains

- >> Constantly worries about everything

- >> Seems terrified by anything specific, such as insects, dogs, driving, thunderstorms, and so on

- >> Responds with irritation when pushed to attend social functions, such as parties, weddings, meetings, neighborhood functions, or anywhere you may encounter strangers (the resistance could be due to simple dislike of the activity, but carefully consider whether anxiety may lie at the root of the problem)

WARNING

A couple of the symptoms in the preceding list (especially irritability, poor concentration, poor sleep, and self-doubts) can also indicate depression. Depression is a serious condition that usually includes loss of interest in activities previously considered pleasurable, changes in appetite, and depressed mood. If your loved one seems depressed, talk with her, and suggest that she consult with a mental health practitioner or her family physician.

Now, if you answered yes to any of the questions in the preceding list, we don't recommend that you approach your loved one and say, "Look at this list — you're a nut case! I knew it." That would be a really bad idea.

TIP

Instead, consider asking your loved one a few questions. This definitely shouldn't occur immediately following a conflict or argument. Possible questions to ask include:

- >> What's the biggest stress in your life lately?

- >> What worries you the most?

- >> Sometimes, when I go to events like this, I feel anxious. I'm wondering how you're feeling about going.

- >> How were you feeling when we left the party?

- >> How are you feeling about that problem?

- >> I've noticed you've had trouble sleeping lately. What's been on your mind?

TIP

Try to make your questions as nonthreatening and safe to answer as possible. In addition, try to ask questions that don't have a simple yes or no answer. For example, if you ask your partner whether she's anxious, she may reply with a simple "No," and then the discussion is over. But if you ask what worries she has, you may get a more complete response. Finally, asking "what" or "how" works better than asking "why" someone is feeling anxious — people often can't answer "why" they feel the way that they do.

Our list of questions for you about your loved one's anxiety and our list of questions to ask your loved one open the door to communicating about anxiety. After you broach the subject, and confirm that the one you care about struggles with anxiety, you can build a plan from there. But you need to know how to keep the conversation going.

WARNING

You don't want to play the role of your loved one's therapist. Even if you're a trained therapist, it's a terrible idea to take that on. Your role should be supportive. If anxiety or other emotional issues are interfering with your loved one's happiness or day-to-day functioning, gently suggest professional help.

Talking Together about Anxiety

Talking about a loved one's vulnerability isn't always easy. Keeping a few ideas in mind may help. For example, if you find the conversation turning into an argument, it's not helpful. Back off. Your loved one may not be ready to face the problem. If so, you may want to check out the "Accepting Anxiety with Love" section later in this chapter.

WARNING

Not every couple communicates easily about difficult subjects without arguing. If that's the case for the two of you, we suggest relationship counseling — reading a few pages about talking together won't solve fundamental communication problems. But if you're able to talk together about anxiety without experiencing a communication breakdown, we have some general guidelines for you in the following sections.

WARNING

If your loved one has a problem with anxiety, you may find yourself feeling oddly ambivalent about helping. Sometimes, those confusing feelings come from the fact that seeing one's partner improve can upset the power balance in a relationship. If you prefer being the boss in your relationship, you may feel uncomfortable seeing your partner get better and become more equal to you. If you see that struggle in yourself, we suggest you seek relationship counseling. You're likely to discover that a more equal relationship feels better than your unconscious mind thinks it will.

Helping without owning the albatross

The first order of business in a discussion of your partner's anxiety is to show empathetic concern. That means putting yourself in your partner's shoes and seeing the world through his eyes. Then, you can try to understand the source of the worry.

However, expressing empathy and concern doesn't mean that you need to solve the problem. You can't. You may be able to help, as we show in the "Guiding the Way" section later in this chapter, but you don't control the emotions of other people — they do.

REMEMBER

Realizing that helpers don't own the responsibility for making change happen is important. Otherwise, you're likely to become frustrated and angry if and when efforts to change stall. Frustration and anger only make overcoming anxiety more difficult.

Avoiding blame

Just as you don't want to blame yourself by owning the problem when your partner becomes anxious, it's equally important to avoid blaming your partner. Your loved one developed anxiety for all the reasons we list in Chapters 3 and 4. Nobody asks for an anxiety disorder. Nobody wants one, and change is difficult.

TIP

People sometimes get upset when they try to help and the response they get consists of resistance and a lack of gratitude. But your loved one may resist your help because anxiety is like an old habit. It may not feel good, but at least it's familiar. When you start to work on reducing anxiety, anxiety typically increases before it gets better.

Therefore, make every effort to avoid blame and be patient. Success and failure aren't up to you. You want to help, but if change doesn't happen, it means nothing about you.

Giving reassurance: When help turns into harm

People with anxiety desperately seek ways to alleviate their distress. One common way is to ask for reassurance. If it's your partner who has anxiety, of course you want to help by giving that reassurance. For example, people who have a great fear of illness often ask their spouses if they look okay or if they're running a temperature. Unfortunately, reassuring your partner makes anxiety increase over time.

TIP

How can something designed to alleviate anxiety create more anxiety? When an anxious person is reassured that everything is okay, it feels very good to have the anxiety decreased for a while. That immediate reduction in anxiety reinforces or rewards the act of seeking assistance. Thus, giving reassurance teaches the recipient to want more reassurance. Rather than depending on his own good sense, the anxious person looks for help from others. Both dependency and anxiety thereby increase.

Asking for reassurance can take many forms. Sometimes, it's hard to spot. In Table 18-1, we give you some examples of reassurance requests and alternative ways to handle them. The first column gives a brief description of the basis for the fear or anxiety and the reassurance request, and the second column gives you an alternative response to offering reassurance.

TABLE 18-1 **Responding to Reassurance Requests**

Ways Your Loved One May Seek Reassurance	New Ways of Responding
Someone who worries excessively greatly fears being late and asks, "Do you think we'll be on time?" or "When will we be there?" or "Do you think that we left enough time for traffic?"	"You never know," or "I can't really predict the future."
A loved one who worries too much about future finances asks, "How will we ever live okay if the stock market crashes five or ten years from now?"	"We talked about the fact that I can't answer questions like that."
A loved one with a fear of crowds asks, "Do you think I'll be able to handle going to the game with you?"	"I don't know; I guess we'll just have to try it and find out."
Someone with a fear of flying asks, "Do you think the weather will be okay for this flight?"	"Gosh, it's pretty hard to predict the weather."
A person who has social anxiety asks, "Will you make sure that I know the names of everyone there?"	"Well, I may not know all the names and I may not always remember them. You can always tell people you've forgotten their name."
A loved one who worries about getting sick asks, "Do you think I may be getting sick?"	"I really don't know. We've talked about me letting you handle this worry."

WARNING

If you've been in the habit of giving your partner frequent, large doses of reassurance, don't suddenly stop without discussing the issue first. Otherwise, your partner is likely to think you've stopped caring. You need to let your partner know, and come to an agreement that eliminating unnecessary reassurance is a good idea. Then, agree that you'll reassure once on any given concern, but when asked repeatedly, you'll simply smile and say, "We agreed that I can't answer that."

TIP

If your loved one is in therapy, be sure that anything you do to help is agreed upon and coordinated with that therapist. Most therapists are happy to see partners for part or all of a session to coordinate plans.

The following anecdote demonstrates how reassurance can aggravate anxiety and how alternative responses can help. At first, James hooks Roberto into feeling overly responsible for his insecurity and anxiety. Roberto provides more and more reassurance, and James keeps getting worse. A psychologist suggests a new response.

> **James and Roberto** have lived together for the past three years. Both graduate students, they lead busy lives. Lately though, James has stopped attending social events, complaining of fatigue. Roberto finds himself going alone and misses James's company.
>
> Roberto receives an announcement that he's the recipient of this year's Departmental Dissertation of the Year Award. Of course, he wants James to attend, but James fears sitting alone and feeling trapped. Roberto reassures James that the auditorium is safe and that he could get out if he needed to by sitting on the aisle. James still resists, so Roberto suggests they get Brenda, a good friend of theirs, to accompany him.
>
> Finally, after considerable cajoling and reassurance, James agrees to go to the event. He spends the time in the audience clinging to Brenda. He feels momentarily comforted by Brenda's presence and reassurances that everything will be okay. But he believes he couldn't have made it through the awards ceremony without her there to hold his hand.
>
> As each new outing comes up, it seems that James requires more reassurance and attention. James withdraws, becoming more isolated, and his anxiety increases.
>
> Then James finally sees a psychologist who suggests enlisting James's friends to help out. He asks them to provide James new, alternative responses to his reassurance-seeking. At the next event, Roberto insists that James go on his own. When James asks Roberto, "Do you think I'll fall apart?" Roberto tells him, "You'll just have to try it and find out."

Initially, Roberto fell into the trap of not only being empathetic but also owning James's problem. His "help" only served to increase James's dependency. James eventually learns to rely on his own resources and feels empowered by doing so.

REMEMBER

Unfortunately, when you own your partner's problem by giving too much reassurance and excessive help, it usually just makes things worse. Dependency, avoidance, and anxiousness all deepen. It's a matter of balance. Give truly needed help and show real concern, but avoid going too far.

Guiding the Way

Assuming you've had a healthy discussion with your partner about her anxiety problem, you may be able to help further. But first, take a look at yourself. If you also wrestle with anxiety, do all that you can for yourself before trying to help with your partner's anxiety.

After you take care of your own anxiety, you may want to consider coaching your partner to overcome her anxiety. A coach is a guide who encourages, corrects, and supports. Part of the job of a coach requires modeling how to handle stress and worry. You can't do a good job of modeling if you're quaking in your boots.

Coaches can help carry out one of the most effective ways of overcoming anxiety: gradual exposure. *Exposure* involves breaking any given fear into small steps and facing that fear one step at a time. If any given step creates too much anxiety, the coach can help devise ways of breaking the task into smaller pieces. The following sections offer points to keep in mind when you're helping a loved one deal with her anxiety.

WARNING

In all but the mildest cases of anxiety, a professional should oversee the coaching process. Be sure to read Chapter 9 for important details about exposure prior to attempting to help your partner carry out an exposure plan. If your partner resists or argues with you, consult a professional. Of course you want to help, but it isn't worth harming your relationship to do so.

WARNING

Professional coaches have emerged in large numbers over the past decade. These people vary widely in their training and experience. You may want to use one of these folks to help carry out an exposure plan, but you don't want one of these people to diagnose an anxiety disorder or design a treatment plan from beginning to end. The only exception to this rule of thumb is a coach who also happens to be a licensed mental health professional.

Coaching the right way

So, exactly how does a coach help a loved one who has problems with anxiety? In most cases, coaches help their loved one carry out exposure tasks. In other cases, coaches simply provide encouragement and support from the sidelines. Our discussion here focuses on the former role.

Generally, your participation in coaching would first come as a suggestion from the therapist working with your loved one. However, you may bring up the possibility yourself. In either case, you only want to serve as a coach if your partner clearly expresses an interest in and a desire for your assistance.

Coaching won't work if your partner doesn't feel ready to tackle her anxiety. Coaching also won't work if your loved one doesn't want your involvement. In fact, the effort could easily harm your relationship if you push your help too hard.

Not everyone is cut out to be a coach. Coaching requires significant patience, compassion, and time. If you don't have those things in abundance, don't agree to be a coach. Perhaps you can help your loved one in other ways, such as by taking on a few extra household tasks or simply by being an interested, supportive bystander.

Assuming you choose to accept the position, coaching requires you to take the following actions to be the best coach you can be:

>> **Define your role:** Come to a clear understanding of how much and what type of input your loved one and her therapist want. Do they want you to be involved in the planning? How so? Ask whether they want you to simply observe the exposure activities or actively encourage carrying out the tasks involved with exposure. Make sure they're specific about what they want you to do. For example, ask whether you should stand next to your partner, hold a hand, or stand a few feet away during exposure tasks.

>> **Encourage while keeping emotions in check:** Because you care so much, it's really easy to let your emotions guide your behavior while you coach. You want to encourage, but do so gently and calmly. Be careful not to

- Push too hard. If your partner says "enough," it's enough.

- Become too enthusiastic about progress. Your partner may feel it as pressure.

- Get angry or argue. Remember to accept whatever your partner is able to do.

- Become tearful or discouraged.

- Feel overly involved with the process.

- Start losing sleep.

If the coaching process causes you to become overly emotional or upset, back off. You may not be the right person for this job. That doesn't mean you don't care; in fact, you may simply care too much to be a good coach.

>> **Avoid excessive responsibility:** Your loved one must develop an exposure plan, usually in concert with a therapist. You may help the one you care about develop a few details of the plan, but don't take on the full responsibility for designing an exposure list. People who have problems with anxiety frequently feel insecure and ask for excessive help and reassurance. Don't be pulled in by your loved one's insecurity.

>> **Stick with the plan:** Resist the temptation to improvise. After a plan is in place, stick to it. If changes need to be made, consult with your loved one or have her discuss it with her therapist. Don't throw in surprises.

>> **Remain positive:** Coaches need to avoid criticism and judgment. Your loved one won't be spurred on by negative comments from you. People work hard for praise and become immobilized and defensive in response to criticism. Avoid saying anything like, "You *should* be able to do this," or "You aren't working hard enough."

>> **Maintain realistic expectations:** After the plan is in place, expect your partner to have ups and downs. Some days go better than others. Small steps eventually go a long way. But you must always remember that determining how the plan plays itself out isn't up to you.

>> **Execute the game plan:** After an exposure plan has been developed, the next step is to begin with relatively easy tasks. A good coach provides support and feedback. In addition, the coach can model, reward, and focus attention. Here are a few additional tips:

- Before asking your loved one to carry out a step, see whether she wants you to model the task first. If you model, showing a small amount of anxiety yourself is fine if you feel it.

- Set up some rewards for success at a few intervals along the exposure list. Do something you can enjoy together. You can also give some honest praise for success; just be sure not to sound patronizing or condescending.

- If the person you care about appears anxious at any step but not overwhelmed, encourage staying with that step until the anxiety comes down. Obviously, don't absolutely insist, just encourage. Remind your partner that anxiety comes down with enough time. And it's not essential for the anxiety to decrease in order for the exposure work to do some good.

Looking at a coach in action

Coaching someone you care about can seem overwhelming. The following example about Doug and Rosie helps you see how one couple worked through a mild case of anxiety with the help of a good game plan.

Doug and Rosie have dated for over a year. In all that time, they've never gone to a movie together because Rosie wrestles with a mild case of agoraphobia (a fear of being trapped and unable to escape). Although she's able to go most places and do what she needs to in life, she dreads going anywhere that makes her feel trapped, especially movie theaters. She fantasizes that she'll need to get out, but she won't find her way to an exit because of the crowd and the darkness. She imagines that she would trip over people, fall on her face, and desperately crawl through the darkened theater.

Doug realizes that Rosie makes one excuse after another to avoid going to movies, even though she enjoys watching them on television. Gently, he asks Rosie, "Some things make me a little anxious — heavy traffic or big crowds — what makes you anxious?" Rosie confesses that crowded movie theaters make her feel closed in and trapped.

Doug and Rosie have a productive discussion about her concerns and decide to face them. Doug is familiar with the concept of exposure and tries to apply the concepts of gradual exposure to Rosie's fear of going to the movies. They discuss the fact that if exposure bogs down, they'll stop the process and seek the input of a professional mental health therapist.

First, together they devise a list, which breaks down the feared situation into small steps. Their list looks like this:

- Going to a short movie with Doug that's not very popular or crowded during an early afternoon while choosing an aisle seat.
- Going to a longer movie that's not crowded with Doug, early afternoon, and sitting on the aisle.
- Same scenario; middle seat.
- Going to an early evening show that's moderately crowded, aisle seat with Doug.
- Same scenario; middle seat.
- Going to an opening for a popular show with Doug, arriving early and choosing an aisle seat.
- Same set up; choosing a middle seat with Doug.

In some cases, an exposure list would include going to a popular, crowded movie by herself. However, Rosie decides she's not particularly interested in being able to watch a movie by herself. So, she chooses to end the exposure exercises with attending a crowded movie in the evening with Doug.

Not only does Doug accompany Rosie to the movies, he also celebrates her successes and encourages her when she starts to falter. He holds her hand on the easier items and gives less support toward the end. Gradually, Rosie feels less anxiety when watching movies with Doug.

They begin enjoying their nights at the movies and find that they both love talking about their experiences afterward over coffee and dessert. She feels good about her accomplishment, and the two of them become closer.

Rosie's fear of the movies had not yet reached the level of severely interfering with her life. Therefore, it was a good choice for a relatively simple exposure plan. Had Rosie not dealt with her fear in this early stage, it would likely have spread from fear of movies to fear of other crowded places.

REMEMBER

Most people with fears and anxieties need to develop a plan with the help of a therapist. However, the example of Rosie and Doug serves as an illustration of how a simple plan sometimes can be carried out without a therapist.

Teaming Up against Anxiety

TIP

One way you can help your partner overcome anxiety is to collaborate on ways to decrease stress in both your lives. With a little ingenuity, you can explore a variety of solutions that are likely to feel good to you even if you personally don't suffer from anxiety at all. For example:

>> **Take a stress management class online or at a local center for adult continuing education.** These classes help people make lifestyle changes and set goals. Many of the ideas make life more fun and interesting in addition to reducing stress.

>> **Take regular walks with your partner.** It's a great way to reduce stress, but even if you don't have much stress, strolling under the sky together is a wonderful time to talk and is great for your health.

>> **Take a yoga, Pilates, or tai chi class together.** Again, even if you don't have anxiety, these classes are terrific for balance, muscle strength, flexibility, and overall health.

>> **Explore spirituality together.** You may choose to attend a church, a synagogue, or a mosque, or scope out a less traditional method of communing with a higher power, such as immersing yourselves in nature. Thinking about things bigger than yourselves or the mundane events of the world provides a peaceful perspective.

>> **Look for creative ways to simplify your joint lives.** Consider looking for help with household chores if you both work. Carefully analyze the way that you spend time. Make sure that your time reflects your priorities.

>> **Do something good.** Consider jointly volunteering for a worthwhile cause or charity. Many people feel that such work enhances the meaning and purpose of their lives. Look at animal shelters, food banks, hospitals, and schools as possibilities. Even an hour every other week can make a positive difference.

>> **Get away.** Take a vacation. You don't have to spend much money. And if you don't have the time for a long vacation, go away for an occasional evening at a local hotel. Getting away from texting, telephones, emails, doorbells, and other endless tasks and demands, even for a night, can help rejuvenate both of you.

Accepting Anxiety with Love

It may seem rather counterintuitive, but accepting your loved one's battle with anxiety is one of the most useful attitudes that you can take. Acceptance paradoxically forms the foundation for change. In other words, whenever you discuss your loved one's anxiety or engage in any effort to help, you need to appreciate and love all your partner's strengths and weaknesses.

You fell in love with the whole package — not just the good stuff. After all, you're not perfect, nor is your loved one. You wouldn't want perfection if you had it. If perfect people even existed, we can only imagine that they would be quite boring. Besides, studies show that people who try to be perfect more often become depressed, anxious, and distressed.

TIP

Therefore, rather than expecting perfection, accept your loved one as is. You need to accept and embrace both the possibility of productive change as well as the chance that your partner may remain stuck. Accepting your partner is especially important when your efforts to help

>> Result in an argument

>> Seem ineffective

>> Aren't well-received by your partner

>> Seem merely to increase your partner's anxiety even after multiple exposure trials

What does acceptance do? More than you may think. Acceptance allows you and your loved one to join together and grow closer, because acceptance avoids putting pressure on the one you care about. Intense expectations only serve to increase anxiety and resistance to change.

Acceptance conveys the message that you will love your partner no matter what. You'll care whether your partner stays the same or succeeds in making changes. This message frees your loved one to

>> Take risks

>> Make mistakes

>> Feel vulnerable

>> Feel loved

REMEMBER

Change requires risk-taking, vulnerability, and mistakes. When people feel that they can safely goof up, look silly, cry, or fail miserably, they can take those risks. Think about it. When do you take risks or try new things? Probably not around an especially critical audience.

Giving up anxiety and fear takes tremendous courage in order to face the risks involved. Letting go of your need to see your partner change helps bolster the courage needed. Letting go of your need includes giving up your ego. In other words, this is not about you.

When you take on the role of a helper, it doesn't mean that your worth is at stake. Of course, you want to do the best you can, but you can't force others to change. Your loved one ultimately must own the responsibility.

IN THIS CHAPTER

» Seeing what's making kids so scared

» Knowing when to worry about your kids' anxiety

» Recognizing the usual anxieties of childhood

» Looking at the most common worries of kids

Chapter **19**

Recognizing Anxiety in Kids

Many adults can recall childhood as being a time of freedom, exploration, and fun. Not too many years ago, kids rode bikes in the street and played outside until dark. Kids walked to school — with other kids.

Now, anxious parents wait with their children at bus stops until they're safely loaded. Parents rarely allow kids to leave the home without adult supervision. Parents worry about predators, kidnappers, pandemics, and violence. They feel understandably protective. However, anxiety spreads from parents to their children. No wonder so many children experience anxiety.

Some anxiety is typical at certain ages. In this chapter, you discover the difference between normal and problematic anxiety in kids. We explain that some childhood fears are completely normal, while others require intervention. Then, we take a look at the symptoms of anxiety that often cluster together. (We devote Chapter 20 to ways you can ease your child's anxiety. If you're concerned about a particular child, we urge you to seek professional diagnosis and treatment.)

Separating Normal from Abnormal

Childhood anxiety has grown to epidemic proportions during the past 40 to 50 years. Recent statistics from the U.S. government indicate that over 7 percent of children ages 3 to 17 have been formally diagnosed with some type of anxiety disorder. Many more suffer from anxiety but have not been identified or treated. About a third of children with anxiety also suffer from depression. And another third of kids with anxiety have significant behavior problems. These issues continue to increase as children are exposed to the realities of the modern world through various forms of the media. It's pretty likely that the recent pandemic will greatly increase the rates of anxiety, depression, and behavior problems among children around the world.

So what's going on? Why do our children experience emotional turmoil? Of course, we all know the complexities and tensions of the world today — longer work hours, rapidly developing technologies, economic stress, violence, social unrest, global threats from climate change, and pandemics. We also suspect that certain types of parenting hold partial responsibility, as we discuss in Chapter 20.

For the moment, what you as a parent need to know is how to distinguish the normal anxieties of childhood from abnormal suffering. Realize that the vast majority of kids feel anxious at various times to one degree or another. After all, one of the primary tasks of childhood is to figure out how to overcome the fears that life creates for everyone. Successful resolution of those fears usually results in good emotional adjustment. You just need to know whether your children's fears represent normal development or a more sinister frame of mind that requires help. Look at Table 19-1 to get an idea of the anxiety that you can expect your children to experience at one time or another during their youth.

TABLE 19-1   **Does Your Child Have an Anxiety Problem?**

Anxiety Problem	When Anxiety Is Normal	When Anxiety Should Go Away
Fear of separation from mother, father, or caregiver	Common between the ages of 6 months and 24 months. Don't worry!	If this continues with no improvement after age 4, then you have some cause for concern.
Fear of unfamiliar adults	Common from 6 to 10 months.	Don't be too concerned unless you see this after 2 or 3 years of age. And don't worry about a little shyness or wariness after that.
Fear of unfamiliar peers	Common from age 2 until around 3 years old.	If this continues without showing signs of reducing after 3 years, you have some cause for concern.

Anxiety Problem	When Anxiety Is Normal	When Anxiety Should Go Away
Fear of animals, darkness, and imaginary creatures	Common between ages 2 and 6 years.	If these fears don't start to decline by 6 years of age, you have cause for concern. Many kids want a night light for a while; don't worry unless it's excessive.
School phobia	Mild to moderate school or day-care phobia is common from ages 3 to 6; it can briefly reappear when moving from elementary to middle school.	This should decline and cause no more than minimal problems after age 6. A brief reemergence at middle school is okay, but it should quell quickly. If not, it's a concern.
Fear of evaluation by others	This fear almost defines adolescence. Most teens worry a fair amount about what others think of them.	It should gradually reduce as adolescence unfolds. But it's not uncommon for it to last through the late teens.

Table 19-1 gives you some general guidelines about so-called normal childhood fears. However, independent of age, if fears seem especially serious and/or interfere with your child's life or schoolwork in a major way, they may be problematic and warrant attention. In addition, other anxiety problems we describe in the section "Inspecting the Most Common Anxieties in Children," later in this chapter, are not particularly normal at any age.

SLEEP TERROR IN CHILDREN

Childhood sleep disorders, one of the most common complaints brought to pediatricians, can disrupt the whole family. Children usually outgrow sleep disorders, such as bedwetting, frequent awakenings, and problems going to sleep.

Sleep terror, especially strange and frightening to parents, is relatively common, occurring among 1 to 6 percent of all kids; the incidence among adults is less than 1 percent. Sleep terror tends to present itself about an hour and a half after going to bed. The child typically sits up suddenly and screams for up to half an hour. During the episode, the child is actually asleep and is difficult to awaken and comfort. Children don't remember their sleep terror in the morning. Sleep terror most often occurs when children are between ages 4 and 10. By the time a child is a teenager, it usually disappears.

Direct treatments for sleep terror are unavailable as yet. But then again, because children don't remember it, sleep terror usually doesn't cause the children who have it any daytime distress. Too little sleep may increase the likelihood of sleep terror, so parents should make sure their children get enough sleep. And stress may also contribute to sleep terror, so parents should attempt to alleviate stress and other anxieties in their children.

WARNING

If you have any doubts about the seriousness of your children's anxiety, you should consider a professional consultation. A mental health counselor or your pediatrician should be well-equipped to handle your questions, quite possibly in a single visit. Anxiety problems sometimes predate other emotional difficulties, so you shouldn't wait to get them checked out.

Reviewing the Most Common Anxieties in Children

Some fear and anxiety are normal for kids. You can probably remember being afraid of the dark, monsters, or ghosts. However, other types of anxiety, though not always rare, do indicate a problem that you should address. We briefly review the more common types of problematic anxiety in kids in the following sections.

Separation anxiety

As we show in Table 19-1, kids frequently worry about separations from their parents when they're as young as 6 months to perhaps as old as 4 years of age. However, significant fear of separation past about the age of 4, accompanied by the following, warrants intervention:

>> Excessive distress when separated from caregivers or anticipating such separation

>> Exorbitant worry about harm to parents or caregivers

>> Obstinate avoidance of school or other activities because of worries about separation

>> Refusal to go to bed without being near a parent or caregiver

>> Frequent nightmares about separation

>> Frequent physical complaints, such as headaches, stomachaches, and so on, when separated from parents

Among the various anxiety problems, separation anxiety is relatively common in kids, but that doesn't mean it's normal. The average age at which it seems to worsen is around 7 to 8 years. The good news is that a large percentage of those with separation anxiety benefit from a bit of help (from a teacher, counselor, or pediatrician) or simply grow out of it after three or four years.

WARNING

The bad news is that quite a few of these kids go on to develop other problems, especially depression. For that reason, we suggest prompt professional intervention if it persists longer than a month or two and interferes with normal life.

The following story about Tyler and his mother Julie illustrates a typical presentation of separation anxiety in the form of a school phobia. Note that school phobia often also includes an element of social phobia (see the section "Problems connecting with others" later in this chapter).

> **Julie** doesn't know what to do about her 7-year-old son, **Tyler.** Every day, she battles with him about going to school. At first, she thinks he's really sick, so she takes him to the pediatrician. After a complete physical, the doctor reassures her that Tyler is healthy. The doctor encourages Julie to send Tyler to school and warns that if she doesn't, Tyler's behavior is likely to escalate.
>
> "My stomach hurts," whines Tyler. "I don't want to go to school."
>
> "Now sweetie, you've missed so many days," soothes Julie, "you really should go today; you're not that sick."
>
> "But my stomach really hurts; it really, really does Mommy." Tyler begins to sob. "Besides, the other kids don't like me."

GETTING BACK TO SCHOOL

School phobia is a relatively common separation anxiety in childhood. The treatment for school phobia involves getting the child back to school as soon as possible. Children with school phobia often have parents who are slightly anxious themselves and care deeply about their kids. The first step is to convince the parents that they must be firm in their commitment to return the child to school.

A good way to calm the child and get him back to school is to allow for one brief contact between parent and child each day for a few weeks. The parent keeps a phone handy. With agreement from the child's teacher, the child receives a get-out-of-class pass (usable only once each day) that allows the child to call his parent. The parent then speaks to the child for only an agreed-upon two minutes. The child is encouraged to save the pass for times of great distress and praised when he doesn't use the pass at all during a day.

This pass, allowing a parental phone call, gradually fades to one call every other day, one call a week, and so on. After the first few days, if the parents and teachers remain supportive and firm, the problem usually vanishes. If this strategy fails, there are many other techniques for overcoming school phobias. Consult a mental health professional who specializes in child anxiety.

"You will go to school today," Julie says firmly, grabbing Tyler by the hand. Tyler plants his feet and pulls away, screaming. Julie can't believe what he's doing. He actually seems terrified; Julie's never seen him behave this way. Frantically, Tyler runs to his bedroom and hides in his closet. Julie finds him huddled, sobbing.

Tyler suffers from school phobia, a common but serious childhood anxiety involving anxiety about both separation from parents and social worries.

Wisely, Julie decides to seek further professional help. Most school counselors have had lots of experience in dealing with school phobias. See the sidebar "Getting back to school" for a typical treatment strategy.

WARNING

Sometimes, what appears to be a school phobia is actually a result of a child having been bullied at school. School counselors and teachers can help sort this out for you. Be sure to ask them to check into this possibility.

Constant worry

Based on what we know today, *generalized anxiety* is fairly common among kids and more common among older kids than younger ones. It most often develops at the onset of puberty or shortly thereafter and is characterized by

>> Excessive anxiety and worry about school, friendships, or family problems

>> Physical symptoms, such as stomachaches, headaches, or loss of appetite

>> Difficulty concentrating and/or irritability

>> Problems sleeping, restlessness, or agitation

Kids with this problem tend to overthink almost everything. They are plagued with thoughts of "what if?" Often, professional guidance is in order.

Phobias

Most young kids at one time or another exhibit fear of the dark or monsters in the closet. So, don't worry if your child has these fears unless the fear becomes so intense that it disrupts daily living in a significant way. The typical age of onset of a *real* phobia (as opposed to the earlier, minor fears) is about age 8 or 9.

When a specific fear becomes intense and exaggerated, the child avoids the particular object or situation. When the fear is of little consequence to the child's life, then there is no need for concern. For example, if your 8-year-old is terrified of sharks and you live in the desert, it's probably not necessary to worry too much about that fear. However, if the child is terrified of buses and has to take the school bus every day, this would be a problem that needs to be solved.

Another common phobia in children is fear of dentists and injections. That's a big problem when kids need routine care. If the child is particularly loud, teary, and fearful, it can lead parents to avoid needed treatment. Fortunately, this is a very treatable condition, usually with behavior therapy, which is covered in Chapter 9.

ANXIETY AND OBSESSIVE-COMPULSIVE DISORDER (OCD)

OCD usually involves some anxiety. In fact, for many years, OCD was considered an anxiety disorder. Many children who have problems with anxiety also have some symptoms of OCD. Often beginning in childhood, OCD develops on average at around age 10. However, it can occur as early as 4 or 5 years of age; boys tend to get it earlier than girls do.

Obsessions are recurring, unwanted thoughts that your child can't stop. Some of the most common obsessions among children include

- Excessive fear of intruders
- Fear of germs
- Fear of illness
- Fixation on certain numbers

Compulsions involve rituals or various behaviors that your child feels compelled to repeat over and over. Common childhood compulsions include

- Arranging objects in a precise manner
- Excessive handwashing (except during a pandemic, when it's a good idea!)
- Hoarding items of little value
- Repeatedly counting stairs, ceiling tiles, and steps taken while walking

Warning: Many children perform a few harmless rituals that involve magical thinking, such as not stepping on sidewalk cracks. However, any child that exhibits serious signs of OCD should be evaluated. It doesn't matter at what age it shows up, because OCD tends not to improve without treatment. The good news is that treatment really works!

Problems connecting with others

Some kids are just plain shy. They're born that way, and relatives often make comments like, "He's just like his dad was at that age." Sometimes, shyness decreases with age, but when shyness swells and causes a child to fearfully avoid social encounters in everyday life, your little one may have a problem.

Extreme social fears don't usually manage to get noticed that much until around 10 years of age. Signs generally appear at a younger age, but parents often have trouble distinguishing them from shyness until then. You can pick up on it sooner if you observe your children carefully. If their fears of unfamiliar peers or adults show no improvement whatsoever by age 4 or so, and it is getting in the way of the child's everyday adjustment, you may want to check with a professional to determine whether the problem is serious.

POST-TRAUMATIC STRESS DISORDER AMONG CHILDREN

Post-traumatic stress disorder (PTSD) was once considered an anxiety disorder. Kids with PTSD do often suffer from considerable anxiety. Although thankfully rather rare in children, PTSD symptoms are slightly different among kids than adults. Like adults, children can get PTSD from abuse, other directly experienced trauma, or being exposed to excessive media representations of trauma. (PTSD among New York City kids spiked after the September 11 terrorist attacks. Fourth and fifth graders were particularly affected.) Also, similar to adults, kids can develop PTSD from witnessing trauma happening to others, such as seeing a parent or loved one severely hurt.

Many children who have lived through natural disasters and traumas, such as fires, hurricanes, or earthquakes, develop an acute stress disorder, also known as *post-traumatic stress syndrome.* The symptoms are similar to PTSD but usually go away without treatment. For children, the loss of a home appears to be particularly traumatic.

Children with PTSD become restless, agitated, irritable, and unfocused. Instead of having nightmares and intrusive thoughts, children may act out their terror in play. They may have bad dreams, but these usually don't have content specifically relevant to the trauma. Like adults, they become anxious and alert to any possible sign of danger. They also tend to overreact to trivial incidents, such as being bumped into or criticized.

Silent anxiety

Some extremely shy children also have difficulty communicating with others. They are generally able to communicate with their parents or caregivers. However, in school or another social setting, they may become almost completely unable to speak. Some kids stand in total silent fear, unable to move or communicate. Others can whisper to some familiar people. These kids typically become extremely socially isolated and should have an evaluation from a professional.

TIP

If you have a concern about your child's communication skills, discuss it with your pediatrician. They are trained in child development. If there is a problem, ask for a referral to a speech pathologist or child development specialist.

Chapter **20**

Helping Kids Conquer Anxiety

W e think it's pretty tough being a kid today. We picked up our grand-daughter at school the other day. Before leaving, we wrote her name on a big sign and placed it on the dashboard. We waited in a line of mini-vans and SUVs for more than 30 minutes while teachers walked around with bull-horns calling out children's names so that the drivers could identify themselves. The children waited like cows in a secure, fenced-in area. Wow, just getting picked up from school can arouse anxiety.

How can parents and other concerned adults help children navigate this complex world without developing anxiety? In this chapter, we give parents and caregivers some guidance on how to prevent anxiety from taking root. But some kids will have anxiety despite parents' best intentions, so we also provide tips on ways to help those kids who do. Finally, we take a look at signs that indicate the possibility that a child needs professional help, who to seek for such help, and what to expect from mental health professionals.

Nipping Anxiety in the Bud

How does anxiety begin? The risk for developing anxiety begins at conception. That's right, studies of twins have demonstrated that almost half of what causes anxiety lies in your genes. However, that's just the beginning. Many other factors come into play, and you can do much about these factors, as we explain in this section.

Early mastery experiences

When a hungry or uncomfortable baby cries out and parents respond by feeding or comforting, the baby experiences a beginning sense of mastery. In other words, what the baby does results in a predictable outcome.

This early opportunity can be repeated thousands of times over the next few years in various ways. For example, the toddler discovers how to use language to make requests that then get rewarded. If parents respond unpredictably and chaotically to an infant's attempts to control his environment, anxiety is likely to increase.

So to decrease the probability of anxiety, responding predictably to young children is imperative. For young infants, parents should respond with reasonable consistency to most of their distress. Later, predictability is still important but should occur only to age-appropriate distress or requests. In other words, you wouldn't want to reinforce a 2-year-old's temper tantrums by caving in.

TIP

As your children grow older, you should provide as many opportunities as possible for them to experience a feeling of mastery. You can do this by

>> Involving them in sports

>> Interesting them in hobbies that require some skill

>> Playing games of skill, such as puzzles or board games (okay, video games too, as long as they are not excessive)

>> Making sure that they have the chance to experience success at school and getting immediate help if they start struggling with their studies

>> Training them to have good manners and social skills

ANXIETY'S BRAIN CHEMISTRY

Recent research at Columbia University explored the effect of the brain chemical serotonin (a neurotransmitter thought to influence mood), which is produced naturally in the body, on the development of anxiety. Experimenters bred mice that lacked important receptors for serotonin, which left them unable to use this important neurotransmitter. They found that mice between 5 and 20 days old without the ability to process serotonin developed mouse anxiety as adults. But when they raised mice with normal serotonin receptors and later depleted the mice of serotonin when they had reached adulthood, the mice didn't develop anxiety.

What does this research have to do with anxious kids? It points to the importance of biological factors in the development of anxiety. Even prenatal and early infantile experiences may affect emotional well-being long into the future. Perhaps treating childhood anxiety early can help to prevent future problems.

More research is needed to understand how all this works. However, we know that biological interventions (such as medications) affect serotonin levels, and it appears that behavioral strategies, such as those described in this book, also alter brain chemistry in productive ways.

Fine-tuning emotions

One of the most important tasks of childhood consists of learning how to control emotions, tolerate frustration, and delay gratification. Again, young infants need prompt gratification. However, with increasing age, the world tends to look unfavorably upon those who demand instant gratification and rejects those who can't keep a reasonable lid on their emotional outbursts.

TIP

You can help your child learn these crucial skills of emotional regulation. Helping children express emotions without letting them run out of control involves a few basic steps:

>> **Validate your children's emotions.** When children feel distressed, anxious, or worried, validate their emotions. You do that by saying,

- "I see that you're a little afraid of . . ."
- "You seem upset about . . ."
- "You seem worried about . . ."

This validating statement should also try to help your children connect the feeling to what's going on. Also, it's always a good idea to ask your child if your observation correctly identified what your child was feeling.

>> **Don't deny your children's feelings.** To the greatest degree possible, don't deny the feeling or try to take it away. In other words, you don't want to say, "You shouldn't be scared," or, worse, "You're not really afraid."

>> **Don't overprotect.** No one likes to see children feel fearful or anxious. However, they need to figure out how to deal with most fears on their own. If you try to solve all their problems or keep them from all worries and danger, you're doing more harm than good.

>> **Help your kids learn to calm down.** You can teach them to take a few slow, deep breaths or count to ten slowly. You can also explain that extreme anxiety and fear will lessen eventually.

>> **Talk to your child about handling difficult emotions.** When your child is frustrated, have discussions about the causes of frustration and how to deal with being upset in constructive ways. Refrain from lecturing.

>> **Praise your children.** When they make efforts to overcome anxieties, praise your kids. However, don't punish them for failing to do so.

>> **Give your children opportunities to learn patience.** Choose some activities that require waiting and taking turns. When required to wait in line, talk to your child about the advantages of learning patience throughout life.

Inoculating against anxiety

Bad experiences with certain situations, activities, animals, and objects sometimes turns into a phobia (irrational, intense fears resulting in excessive avoidance). These experiences may be real, imaginary, or portrayed in a movie or television show. The following list of children's fears shows that children acquire fears that are often similar to those that adults experience:

>> Airplanes

>> Being alone

>> Dogs

>> Heights

>> Rodents

>> Snakes

>> Spiders and insects

>> Thunder and lightning

TIP

If you want to prevent your children from acquiring one of these common phobias, you can inoculate them. You do that by providing safe interactions with the potentially feared event or object — prior to any fear developing. Try the following activities:

>> Take your kids to a museum or zoo that offers hands-on experiences with snakes and insects.

>> Climb a mountain together.

>> Watch a storm from the safety of your living room couch. Discuss how lightning and thunder work.

>> If you don't have a dog or cat of your own, go to the pound and visit puppies and kittens.

Research has proven that this method works. For example, studies have shown that children bitten by dogs don't develop a phobia as readily if they have had past, positive experiences with dogs. Children who fly at an early age rarely develop a phobia of flying. The more experiences you provide your children with, the better their chances are of growing up without phobias.

TIP

If you're somewhat phobic yourself, try not to make faces or get too squeamish when you inoculate your kids against phobias. Don't say, "Oooh, how gross!" Even if you feel nervous, try not to show it.

Resisting the desire to comfort and reassure

When your kids are frightened, it's natural to feel like comforting them. You want to remove their fears and tell them everything will be alright. We have some surprising advice: *For the most part, we urge you to resist the temptation to reassure your kids when they feel anxious or afraid.*

That's because when you give that reassurance, they feel better. So far, so good. But the next time they feel a bit anxious or afraid, they're likely to ask for more reassurance instead of coping on their own. Unfortunately, when kids seek and receive immediate reassurance, they miss the opportunity to face their fears and develop mature coping skills. And if you, as the parent, are not around to comfort them, they may become overwhelmed with fear, unable to manage their emotions.

REMEMBER

Don't provide unnecessary reassurance. Making comments such as, "There's nothing to be afraid of" is unnecessary. Kids need to find out how to handle a little stress and anxiety on their own. Don't constantly reassure them, or you'll create a surefire path to anxiety.

Taking precautions via parenting style

Parents can set children up to develop an anxiety disorder, or parents can help to prevent anxiety, depending on their parenting style:

>> **Permissive parents** engage with their kids and show concern and caring. But permissive parents hate confrontation, and they abhor seeing their kids feel bad. Therefore, they set low expectations for their children, and they don't push them to act mature or try new things.

>> **Authoritarian parents** represent the opposite extreme. They demand, direct, and expect instant obedience from their children. They control every detail of their children's lives and tend to be overly structured and hostile.

>> **Authoritative parents** take the middle road. These parents set reasonable limits and boundaries. They're flexible and aware of their kids' developmental stage. They try to help their kids understand the reasons behind their expectations for good behavior, although they don't spend a whole lot of time *reasoning,* or debating, with their kids.

Keep reading for more details about how each of these parenting styles affects a child's anxiety level.

Permissive and authoritarian parenting

Both the permissive and the authoritarian types of parents fuel anxiety in children. The following story is about both types. The mother demonstrates permissive parenting, and the father is an authoritarian.

Six-year-old **Nancy** screams with terror. Her parents rush into her room to see what's wrong. "There's a bad man in my room; I saw him," she cries.

Nancy's mother hugs her, strokes her hair, and tells her, "Everything will be okay now that Mommy's here."

Her dad turns on the light. He checks her closet and under her bed and snaps, "There's nobody here. Just stay in your bed, and go to sleep. Don't be such a baby."

When this scene reenacts itself night after night for six weeks, Nancy's dad becomes increasingly annoyed and speaks harshly to her about what he calls her silly fears. At the same time, her mother overprotects Nancy. Her mom even starts to sleep in her room to make her feel safe. Her fears only intensify. Poor Nancy receives mixed messages from her parents, and neither message helps.

Authoritative parenting

TIP

A different kind of parenting can help your kids deal with anxiety better. It's called *authoritative* (as opposed to authoritarian) parenting. Authoritative parents provide clear expectations for their children. They encourage their kids to face challenges. They validate their children's feelings of anxiety but urge them to deal with them. They aren't harsh or punitive, but they don't overprotect. Using Nancy's story again, the following demonstrates how authoritative parents would deal with Nancy's anxieties.

> Six-year-old **Nancy** screams with terror. Her parents rush into her room to see what's wrong. "There's a bad man in my room; I saw him," she cries.
>
> Nancy's mom gives her a quick hug and says, "You sound afraid, sweetie."
>
> Her dad turns on the light, checks the closet and under the bed, and says, "Nobody's here, honey. But if you'd like, we can leave a night light on."
>
> Nancy says, "Please don't leave me alone. Can't Mommy just stay here with me tonight?"
>
> Nancy's mom tells her, "No, you need to handle this yourself. I know you're worried, but it will be okay." They turn the night light on and tell her, "Here's your bear; he'll keep you company. We'll see you in the morning."
>
> Nancy cries softly for a few minutes and falls back to sleep.

Nancy's parents were lucky that she only cried for a short period of time. They felt a bit guilty for letting her cry but realized that Nancy needs to learn that she can handle a little anxiety on her own. Some kids aren't so easy.

Perhaps your child keeps on crying and won't stop. Well, sometimes that happens. Occasionally, you may need to hang in there for an hour or two. The first night is usually the worst. Don't give up. Eventually, the vast majority of kids start falling asleep sooner. If that doesn't happen after four or five nights in a row, you may need to consult a professional.

HELICOPTER PARENTING

Think of a helicopter hovering over you, following you throughout each day as you go about your business. Specifically, *helicopter parents* direct their kids' lives, run interference for them whenever they can, and try to shield them from all bad feelings. Thus, a helicopter parent will complain to teachers about grades or assignments, argue with coaches, and confront their children's peers when a conflict occurs.

It's bad enough when helicopter parents hover in this manner during elementary school. But some of these folks never stop. They continue to prevent their teens from experiencing the consequences of their own behavior and misjudgments. Some of these parents even write their kids' college papers for them. In fact, a few colleges have found that parental interest is so intense that parent-teacher associations (PTAs) have sprung up on college campuses.

Helicopter parents often have high expectations of their kids, unlike permissive parents. However, they're similar to permissive parents in that they can't stand seeing their kids feel frustrated or upset. The problem with both types of parents is that they fail to teach their kids how to deal with life's difficulties. Anxiety often results.

Helping Already Anxious Children

If you have a child with anxiety, don't make yourself anxious by blaming yourself for the problem. Multiple factors probably went into making your kid anxious (for more information, read Chapter 3). And, you probably weren't able to read this book prior to your child developing anxiety, so you didn't know what you could do to prevent it. So now what do you do? Read on.

Helping yourself first

If you've traveled on a commercial flight, you've probably heard flight attendants instruct you about how to deal with the oxygen masks should they drop down. They tell you to put the mask on yourself prior to assisting your child. That's because if you don't help yourself first, you won't be in any condition to help your child.

TIP

The same principle applies to anxiety in your kids. You need to tackle your own anxiety prior to trying to help your children. Children learn many of their emotional responses by observing their parents; it makes sense that anxious parents more often end up with anxious children. The nice part of getting rid of your own anxiety first is that this is likely to help your children, as well as give you the resources for assisting with their worries.

You can do this by reading this book. Pick and choose the strategies that best fit your problem and personality. However, if the ideas you choose first don't seem to work, don't despair. The vast majority of the time, one or more of the techniques that we describe do help.

WARNING

If you find that reading this book and trying our recommendations don't reduce your anxiety as much as you'd like, consider consulting a mental health professional who's trained in cognitive behavioral therapy.

Modeling mellow

If you don't have a problem with anxiety, or if you've overcome your excessive worries for the most part, you're ready to teach by example. Children learn a great deal by watching the people they care about. You may recall a time when your child surprised you by repeating words you thought or wished he hadn't heard. Trust us, kids see and hear everything.

TIP

Therefore, take advantage of every opportunity to model relatively calm behavior and thinking. Don't invalidate your child's anxiety by saying it's a stupid or silly fear. Furthermore, demonstrating complete calm is not as useful as showing how you handle the concern yourself. Table 20-1 shows some common childhood fears and how you can model an effective response.

TABLE 20-1   Modeling a Better Way

Fear	Parental Modeling
Thunderstorms	"I understand a thunderstorm is coming tonight. Sometimes, I get a little nervous about them, but I know we're safe at home. I'm always careful to seek shelter during a thunderstorm. But I know that thunderstorms can't really hurt you when you're inside."
Insects	"I used to think that insects were gross, awful, and scary, but now I realize that they're more afraid of me than I am of them. Insects run away from people when they can. Sometimes, they're so scared that they freeze. I admit that I still use plenty of tissue to pick them up, and that's okay. Let me show you how I do it."
Heights	"I sometimes feel a little nervous looking down from high places. Here we are on the top of the Washington Monument. Let's hold hands and go to the window together. You can't fall off, and it can't hurt you. Looking down from heights is kind of fun. The scariness is kind of exciting after you get used to it."
Being alone (don't say this unless your child expresses anxiety about feeling safe alone)	"Your father's going on a trip tomorrow. I used to feel afraid staying at home by myself, but I realize that I can take pretty good care of myself and of you. We have a security door, and if anyone tries to get in, we can always call the police. Our dogs are pretty good protection, too. Do you ever get scared? If you do, we can talk about it."

Leading children through anxiety

As we discuss in Chapter 9, gradual exposure to whatever causes anxiety is one of the most effective ways of overcoming fear. Whether the anxious person is a child or an adult, the strategy is much the same. Therefore, if you want to help your children who already have anxiety, first model coping as we describe in Table 20-1. Then, consider using *exposure*, which involves breaking the feared situation or object into small steps. You gradually confront and stay with each step until your child feels a bit better.

REMEMBER

Read Chapter 9 for important, additional details about exposure. However, keep a few things in mind when doing this as a guide for your child:

>> **Break the steps down as small as you possibly can.** Don't expect your child to master a fear overnight. It takes time. And children need smaller steps than adults. For example, if you're dealing with a fear of dogs, don't expect your child to immediately walk up to and pet a dog on the first attempt. Instead, start with pictures and storybooks about dogs. Then progress to seeing dogs at a distance, behind an enclosed fence. Gradually work up to direct contact, perhaps at a pet store.

>> **Expect to see some distress.** This is the hard part for parents. No one likes to see their kids get upset. But you can't avoid having your kids feel modest distress if you want them to get over their anxiety. Sometimes, this part is more than some parents can handle. In those cases, a close friend or relative may be willing to pitch in and help. At the same time, if your child exhibits extreme anxiety and upset, you need to break the task down further or get professional help.

>> **Praise your child for any successes.** Pay attention to any improvement and compliment your child. However, don't pressure your child by saying that this shows what a big boy or girl he or she is.

>> **Show patience.** Don't get so worked up that your own emotions spill over and frighten your child further. Again, if that starts to happen, stop for a while, enlist a friend's assistance, or seek a professional's advice.

The following story shows how parents dealt with their son's sudden anxiety about water. Kids frequently become afraid when something unexpected happens.

> **Penny and Stan** plan a Caribbean vacation at a resort right on the beach. The brochure describes a family-friendly atmosphere. They purchase a snorkel and diving mask for their 3-year-old, **Benjamin,** who enjoys the plane ride and looks forward to snorkeling.

When they arrive, the hotel appears as beautiful as promised. The beach beckons, and the ocean water promises to be clear. Penny, Stan, and Benjamin quickly unpack and make their way down to the beach. They walk into the water slowly, delighted by the warm temperature. Suddenly, a large wave breaks in front of them and knocks Benjamin over. Benjamin opens his mouth in surprise, and saltwater gags him. He cries and runs back to the shore, screaming.

Stan immediately pulls Benjamin back into the water. He continues to scream and kick. Penny and Stan spend the rest of the vacation begging Benjamin to go into the ocean again to no avail. The parents end up taking turns babysitting Benjamin while their vacation dream fades.

At home, Benjamin's fear grows, as untreated fears often do. He fusses in the bath, not wanting any water to splash on his face. He won't even consider getting into a swimming pool.

Benjamin's parents take the lead and guide him through exposure. First, on a hot day, they put a rubber, inflated wading pool in the backyard. They fill it and model getting in. Eventually, Benjamin shows a little interest and joins them in the pool. After he gets more comfortable, the parents do a little playful splashing with each other and encourage Benjamin to splash them. He doesn't notice that his own face gets a little water on it.

Then his parents suggest that Benjamin put just a part of his face into the water. He resists at first, but they encourage him. When he puts his chin into the water, they applaud. Stan puts his face entirely under water and comes up laughing. He says that Benjamin may not be ready to do that. Benjamin proves him wrong. Benjamin and Stan take turns putting their faces into the water and splashing each other. What started out as fear turns into fun.

The parents provide a wide range of gradually increasing challenges over the next several months, including using the mask and snorkel in pools of various sizes. Then they go to a freshwater lake and do the same. Eventually, they take another vacation to the ocean and gradually expose Benjamin to the water there as well.

If Benjamin's parents had allowed him to play on the beach at the edge of the water instead of insisting that he get back in the water immediately, he may have been more cooperative. They could have then gradually encouraged him to walk in the water while watching for waves. That way, they may have been able to enjoy their vacation. They made the mistake of turning a fear into a power struggle, which doesn't work very well with children — or, for that matter, with adults.

Exorcizing anxiety through exercise

Exercise burns off excess adrenaline, which fuels anxiety. All kids obviously need regular exercise, and studies show that most don't exercise enough. Anxious kids may be reluctant to engage in intense physical activities like hiking, jogging, biking, or organized sports. They may feel inadequate or even afraid of negative evaluation by others.

REMEMBER

Yet, it may be more important for anxious kids to participate in sports or other physical activities for two reasons. First, these activities provide them with important mastery experiences. Although they may feel frustrated and upset at first, they usually experience considerable pride and a sense of accomplishment as their skills improve. Second, aerobic activity directly decreases anxiety.

TIP

The challenge is to find an activity that provides your child with the greatest possible chance of at least modest success. Consider the following:

>> **Swimming:** An individual sport that doesn't involve balls thrown at your head or collisions with other players. Swimmers compete against themselves, and many swim teams reward most participants with ribbons, whether they come in first or sixth.

>> **Hiking:** This can be done with organized groups or as a family outing. Difficulty can be low, medium, or intense. Kids can learn about how to handle weather emergencies and what supplies they need. They can acquire mastery skills by learning about dangerous plants and creatures.

>> **Track and field:** An individual sport that has a wide variety of different skill possibilities. Some kids are fast and can run short dashes. Others discover that they can develop the endurance to run long distances. Still others can throw a shot put.

>> **Tennis:** A low-contact and relatively safe sport. Good instruction can make most kids adequate tennis players.

>> **Martial arts:** Good for enhancing a sense of competence and confidence. Many martial arts instructors have great skill for working with uncoordinated, fearful kids. Almost all kids can experience improvements and success with martial arts.

>> **Dance:** A sport that includes many variations, from ballet to square dancing. Musically inclined kids often do quite well with dance classes.

In other words, find something for your kids to do that involves physical activity. They can benefit in terms of decreased anxiety, increased confidence, and greater connections with others. Don't forget to include family bike rides, camping trips, and walks. Model the benefits of lifelong activity and exercise.

Getting Help from Others

The goals of childhood include learning how to get along with others, developing self-control, and preparing for adult responsibilities. Children make progress toward these goals by interacting with friends and family as well as by attending school. If anxiety interferes with these activities, then consultation and professional treatment may be needed. In other words, if a child can't play, learn, or participate in activities because of worries, it's time to get help.

Who to get help from

We recommend that parents first turn to their child's medical doctor to make sure there are no physical reasons for a child's anxiety. Certain medications prescribed for other conditions can cause a child to feel anxious. The physician may decide to switch medications first. If the culprit is anxiety, rather than a drug or physical problem, the medical provider may have recommendations for mental health providers. The following tips may help you search more effectively:

>> **Call your health insurance plan to see what type of coverage you have for your child's mental health care.** Your company may have a list of providers in your area.

>> **Call providers and ask whether they have experience and training in treating childhood anxiety.** The therapy can seem like play to your child, but therapy should be based on an approach that has been shown to help children overcome anxiety. We generally recommend practitioners trained in cognitive or behavioral strategies because their effectiveness has been supported most consistently by research.

>> **Make sure the provider you choose has office hours that can accommodate several appointments.** Although the treatment may be relatively brief, don't expect it to happen in one or two sessions.

>> **Ask what state license your provider holds.** Don't seek help from someone without a license to practice mental health counseling. Professionals who usually treat children may be clinical psychologists, social workers, counselors, or school psychologists.

WARNING

Psychiatrists can also be involved in treating childhood anxiety disorders; however, they usually prescribe medication. We recommend that treatment for anxiety, especially for children, begin with psychotherapy rather than medication. We take this approach because of unknown side effects of long-term use of medication and the great potential of relapse when medication is stopped. In contrast, the new ways of thinking and behaving learned through psychotherapy can last a lifetime.

Research has shown that medical costs of anxious children run much higher than costs for kids without anxiety. Covering effective treatment for anxious children is cost-effective for health insurance companies. Your medical provider may be able to advocate with your insurance company using this argument. Treating anxiety early can save considerable money and suffering in the long run.

What to expect at the first session

Generally, the first session is a time for your child's therapist to find out about the problems your child is having. You can expect lots of questions. Parents are almost always invited into the first session to provide information. You may want to prepare for the first appointment beforehand by keeping a journal of what you're concerned about. For example, consider taking notes on the following questions:

>> **What happens?** Does your child avoid certain situations? Is anxiety getting in the way of her schoolwork or play with other children? Is she getting bullied at school?

>> **When do your child's symptoms crop up?** Is he fine at home with familiar people and afraid at school? Does he get worse when he's worried about a test or when meeting new people? Are there particular times when his anxiety seems better or worse?

>> **How long have you noticed these symptoms?** Have there been any changes in the family, such as the birth of a child, death, or divorce? Has your child experienced any trauma?

>> **Do other members of the family have problems with anxiety?** If so, what sorts of problems?

>> **Has your child experienced any recent health problems or hospitalizations?**

Generally, what a parent or child says to a therapist is held in strict confidence with only a few limitations. One important limit to confidentiality with professionals is that they're required to report suspicions of child abuse. Another limit is that they must report cases involving children who appear to represent an imminent threat of harm to themselves or other people.

What happens in therapy?

For young children, much of the work is likely to focus on the parents. In other words, the therapist spends much of the time teaching the parents things they can do to facilitate their child's progress. This focus doesn't mean the parents caused the problem, but they often can do much to alleviate it.

Older children and teenagers spend more time in discussions with the therapist, and parents' involvement varies more widely. In either case, you can expect the therapist to give tasks to both parents and kids to be carried out in between sessions. You should expect the therapist to discuss what the specific goals of the sessions are, as well as detailed plans for getting there. However, you shouldn't expect therapists to reveal details of what is discussed in sessions with your child. Kids need to feel safe in revealing whatever they want to their therapists. Parents are, however, entitled to progress updates.

More often than not, childhood anxiety can be expected to improve significantly (not necessarily resolve entirely) within six months or so of treatment. If that doesn't seem to be happening, discuss it with the therapist and consider getting a second opinion.

6

The Part of Tens

Chapter **21**

Ten Approaches That Just Don't Work

I t's tempting to look for quick and easy ways to beat anxiety; after all, anxiety doesn't feel that great. However, certain thoughts or behaviors can actually make your anxiety worse, do nothing for you, or even waste your hard-earned money. This chapter steers you away from ten approaches to anxiety management that simply don't work.

Avoiding What Makes You Anxious

Avoiding what scares you actually works! But only briefly; then it fuels anxiety. Anxiety intensifies and burns out of control. For example, say you're afraid of driving during rush hour in bumper-to-bumper traffic. So, even though it takes you twice as long, you find slow-moving side roads as an alternative. Your anxiety decreases.

But, the longer you avoid what you fear, the worse it seems. You start noticing increased traffic and faster cars on the slow roads — actually, the traffic is the same, but you're becoming more sensitive to it. So, you look for an even slower route that takes even longer. Your anxiety lessens, but then increases again. That's how avoidance works — in truth, how avoidance *doesn't* work to reduce your anxiety.

Whining and Complaining

It's not fair that you have a problem with anxiety. You didn't ask for it. You could be tempted to complain and whine about your plight. Some people think whining helps because, in the short run, expressing such feelings feels like a release, what's often called "venting."

However, whining and complaining solve nothing. Furthermore, you won't make a lot of friends by wallowing in self-pity — after a while, people grow weary of hearing endless complaining. Managing anxiety requires taking action. You can find lots of ways to take productive actions throughout this book.

Seeking Comfort

Everyone needs a hug sometimes. People enjoy being comforted by friends and family. Enjoy your hugs! Just don't use soothing from others as a way to deal with your anxiety. Unfortunately, the short-term costs of comforting reassurance far outweigh the benefits. Overcoming anxiety requires a willingness to embrace and experience the very situations that make you feel uncomfortable.

TIP

The more you allow anxiety to come in and stay a while, the easier it gets to handle your fears.

Looking for a Quick Fix

Everyone likes instant gratification. You can find almost anything you want online in seconds, whether it be stuff or information. And most people are accustomed to receiving items on their doorsteps in days or even hours. You may be greatly annoyed at delays, glitches, or errors that disrupt that instant gratification.

No wonder people want quick fixes for emotional upsets. Anxiety feels bad, so it's tempting to search for an immediate fix. Sort of like the convenience we all imagine from a meal delivery service — delicious, healthy, pre-prepared, microwaveable dinners. However, like quick fixes for anxiety, the reality is usually a bit disappointing.

Sipping Herbal Tea

Nothing wrong with drinking a cup of tea when you feel anxious. Hold the cup in your hands, breathe in the warm scent, and enjoy the comfort of sipping and sitting quietly. And your anxiety may even decrease some for a few minutes.

If you can manage your schedule such that you sit around all day by yourself sipping tea, that could be a good plan! But most people don't have the luxury of sitting around all day sipping tea. And then there's the problem of boredom, which just might be worse than the anxiety. So, enjoy your cup of tea, but work on your anxiety, too.

Drowning Your Sorrows

Anxiety is a risk factor for substance abuse. People who feel anxious in social situations are at an especially high risk. That's because some substances make people less inhibited, less anxious, and able to talk more freely to others.

Once again, though, the issue of short-term versus long-term gains comes into play. Substances such as alcohol may loosen the tongue, numb your uncomfortable feelings, and feel good in the moment. But the long-term consequences of dependency and abuse far outweigh the momentary benefit of having a good time at a party. If you have social anxiety, consider getting professional help, especially if you're using substances to cope.

Trying Too Hard

Don't get anxious about ridding yourself of anxiety. We're glad you're here to get some advice and suggestions, but it took you a while to get here, didn't it? Rushing the process inadvertently slows progress. Slow down, and enjoy the ride. You'll get there more surely if you don't try to set speed records.

Hoping for Miracles

Hope is good. Miracles can happen. You have to decide how long you're willing to wait around, hoping for a miracle to show up, though. Possibly a better plan is to pray for a miracle but put in your own effort during your wait.

You can become your own solution by facing your anxiety problem and moving forward with mastering skills and coping strategies. Acceptance of feelings, working through thoughts, and trying on new behaviors will help you achieve your own miracle.

Taking Medication as a Solution

Some medications help *some* people with *some* anxiety problems, *some* of the time. But many anti-anxiety medications have a high potential for abuse and addiction. Discuss this issue in depth with your primary care provider (PCP) before taking them. Other medications such as antidepressants can be useful to treat certain types of anxiety with less potential for abuse. See Chapter 10 for more detail and an analysis of the pluses and minuses of other medication options.

REMEMBER

The strategies and therapies described in this book have proven to be more reliable and effective in the long run than medications. Even if your PCP suggests that you consider medication for anxiety, cognitive behaviorally based psychotherapy will likely be more beneficial.

Getting Help on the Couch

You may wonder why we include getting help on the couch in this list of what doesn't work. After all, we have consistently suggested that psychotherapy is an effective treatment for anxiety. But all psychotherapies are not alike.

The type of therapy known for lying on the couch refers to psychoanalysis. Although psychoanalysis-based therapy has shown effectiveness for certain types of problems, it's efficacy for anxiety problems is more questionable.

Chapter **22**

Ten Ways to Deal with Relapse

I f you're reading this chapter, you've probably made some headway with your anxiety. Maybe, after all your hard work, you've experienced a setback, or perhaps you're worried about one. Not to worry. We have ten ideas for you to use when anxiety shows up again in your life.

Expecting Anxiety

Perhaps you've worked hard to overcome your anxiety, and now your hard work has paid off. You've beaten it. Congratulations! But alas, one day you wake up suddenly with anxiety staring you in the face. You turn it into a catastrophe and assume that you've failed.

Oh, get real. You'll never totally annihilate anxiety. That is, until you stop breathing. It's bound to show up from time to time. *Expect* anxiety. Look for its early warning signs. But don't compound matters by getting anxious about your anxiety. If you understand that anxiety happens, you can lessen the impact.

Counting the Swallows

The proverb "One swallow doesn't make a summer" reflects the fact that a single sign doesn't necessarily indicate that something more is inevitable. The arrival of a lone bird doesn't mean the whole flock is back for the season. Anxiety has an ebb and flow. Having an anxious episode or two doesn't mean that you're back to square one. You figured out how to handle some of your anxiety, and that knowledge can still help you. You don't need to start all over again. You do need to move forward, and reapply what you practiced. Thinking of minor setbacks as catastrophes will only increase your anxiety and immobilize your efforts. Regroup, reorganize, and go back at it!

Checking Out Why Anxiety Returned

Minor relapses are a great opportunity to discover what gives you trouble. Figure out what events preceded your latest bout of anxiety:

>> Have you had some recent difficulties at work, such as deadlines, promotions, problems with co-workers, or financial setbacks?

>> Have you had recent problems at home, such as divorce, problems with a child, or other stressors?

If so, understand that an increase in your anxiety is a natural response and likely to be temporary. Use the new information about your anxiety triggers to challenge your anxious thinking, or work on accepting a little bit of anxiety into your life.

Seeing a Doctor

If you've looked high and low for situations or events that may have set off your relapse and can't come up with anything at all, consider making an appointment with your primary care physician. Anxiety can have a number of physical causes, such as side effects from prescription medication or over-the-counter medications and supplements, excessive caffeine, and other health problems (which are covered in Chapter 3). Don't try to diagnose yourself. If you experience anxiety with absolutely no apparent cause, please check it out with your primary care provider.

Revisiting What Worked Before

If anxiety creeps back into your life, review the strategies that worked for you previously. Some of those techniques may need to become lifelong habits. Keep relaxation in your life. Exercise on a regular basis.

REMEMBER

Anxiety isn't a disease that you can cure with a one-time injection, pill, or surgery. Anxiety is a natural part of life. When it mushrooms to a distressing degree, you merely need to reapply the strategies that worked for you.

Doing Something Different

We've presented a variety of strategies for overcoming anxiety. Most likely, you've picked a few that have felt compatible with your lifestyle. Now, consider looking at some ideas you haven't yet attempted. We urge you to do something different. Take a look at the list that follows, and choose one you haven't gotten around to trying yet:

>> Rethinking your anxiety (see Chapters 6 and 7)

>> Facing fear head-on (see Chapter 9)

>> Accepting anxiety (see Chapter 8)

>> Exercising and getting a good night's sleep (see Chapter 11)

If you've simply dabbled at one or more of these techniques, pursue it more aggressively, and see whether it works better that way. Anything in this book that you haven't tried yet is worth considering.

Getting Support

You don't have to face anxiety relapses alone. Talking with others helps you deal with emotional distress. A great source of such support can be found in self-help groups listed in your local newspaper. Perhaps your place of worship has an adult group for people dealing with emotional challenges. You may have a special trusted friend to talk things over with, but be careful not to be too burdensome or one sided in your relationship.

TIP

But what if you live in Pie Town, New Mexico: population 93? Pie Town may not have an anxiety support group. But all is not lost. You can search online for "chat rooms for anxiety." You'll find more than enough interesting sources of support. Try out a few, and see whether you can find a group that feels compatible. Millions of people suffer from anxiety, and they have great advice and support to offer you. You don't need to suffer alone.

REMEMBER

The best support groups give you ideas for coping. Beware of groups that seem to encourage whining and complaining. Also, be very careful of sharing personal information online.

Considering Booster Sessions

If you've seen a professional and later experience an unexpected increase in your anxiety, think about calling for a few booster sessions. Your therapist isn't going to think you failed. Usually, a second round of therapy helps and doesn't take as long as the first. In addition, some people like to check in every few weeks or months as a kind of prevention. Again, anxiety isn't a disease with a single, one-shot cure.

On the other hand, if you've never seen a professional and you experience a relapse, you should consider it now. If you've had previous success on your own, you're likely to improve rapidly with a little assistance.

Doubling Down on Exposure

Consider a return of anxiety an opportunity to practice exposure. Exposure, as we cover in Chapter 9, involves facing your fears until they become less intense. Avoidance of anxiety guarantees that anxiety will only persist and usually grow. So, when you experience a relapse of anxiety, try to welcome it as a potentially positive lesson in developing solid tools for growth.

Accepting Anxiety

With this tip, we come full circle — back to the top of the list: Anxiety happens. It will return. Welcome it with open arms. It means that you're still alive! Appreciate the positive aspects. Anxiety tells you to pay attention to what's going on around you. Go with the flow.

REMEMBER

We're not suggesting that you need to feel horrendous amounts of anxiety, but a little anxiety is unavoidable. And anxiety, when not overwhelming, may help mobilize your resources during difficult challenges.

Chapter **23**

Ten Signs That You Need Professional Help

S ome people find that self-help is all they need. They read about good ways of dealing with their anxiety, and then they apply what they've discovered. Voilà! Their anxiety gradually fades to a manageable level.

However, no self-help book is intended to completely replace professional help. And anxiety sometimes requires the assistance of a professional, just like complicated tax matters may call for a certified public accountant or deciding to draw up a will may send you to an attorney. We hope you understand that seeking a mental health professional's assistance is a reasonable choice, not a sign of weakness.

This chapter tells you how to know whether you should consider professional assistance for yourself or someone you care about. It's not always an obvious decision, so we give you a list of indicators. And if you still aren't sure, you can always talk with your primary care doctor, who should be able to help you decide.

Having Suicidal Thoughts or Plans

If you find yourself thinking about harming yourself, get help now. Take these thoughts very seriously. Call the national suicide hotline at 1-800-273-TALK (1-800-273-8255). If your thoughts become overwhelming, call 911, and get to an emergency room. Help is available. And when you do access professional help, be honest about your thoughts; hold nothing back. A professional can help gather other options and solutions that seem out of reach when someone is feeling tremendously anxious or depressed.

Feeling Hopeless

From time to time, everyone feels defeated. But if you begin to feel hopeless about getting better, thinking that the future looks bleak, and you can't do much to change it, get professional help. Feelings of hopelessness put you at greater risk for suicide. You need to know that you can feel better. Let others help you.

Handling Anxiety and Depression

You may be experiencing depression mixed with anxiety if you find yourself having some of the following symptoms:

» Feeling sad most of the day

» Losing interest or pleasure in activities

» Change in weight

» Changes in your sleep patterns and habits

» Decreased interest in sex

» Feeling keyed up or slowed down

» Feeling worthless

» Feeling excessively guilty

» Poor concentration

» Thoughts of death

If you do have both anxiety and depression, seek professional help. Depression is a treatable condition. Having the energy to fight both can be hard.

Trying to No Avail

Perhaps you've read this book and given the recommendations your best shot at overcoming anxiety, but for whatever reason, they just haven't worked. That's okay. Don't get more anxious because you didn't get rid of worry and stress. Something else may be going on. Get an experienced mental health professional to help you figure out the next step.

Struggling at Home

You're anxious. The anxiety causes you to be irritable, jumpy, and upset. You hold it together at work and with strangers, but you take it out on the people you care about most, your family. Then you feel guilty, which increases your anxiety. If this sounds like you, a professional may help you decrease the tension at home and ease the pathway to finding peace.

Dealing with Major Problems at Work

Maybe you have no one at home to take out your anxiety on, or perhaps home is the haven away from stress. If that's the case, work stress may overwhelm you. If you find your anxiety exploding at work, consider professional help.

First, anxiety sometimes causes irritability and moodiness with co-workers or bosses; such behavior can cause plenty of trouble. Anxiety can also rob you of your short-term memory, make it difficult to focus, or make decisions feel overwhelming. So if anxiety affects your job performance, get help before you hit the unemployment line.

On the other hand, if you're out of work, take a look at Chapter 14 for ideas.

Suffering from Severe Obsessions or Compulsions

Anxiety is a problem that often co-occurs with other emotional disorders. *Obsessive-compulsive disorder* (OCD) is one of those disorders. OCD can easily consume many hours of time and cause serious impairment in the lives of those who suffer from it. The problem is that people with the disorder often don't seek help until their lives are overwhelmed by unwanted thoughts or repetitive actions. Most people with OCD need professional help. If you, or someone you love, has more than mild OCD, get professional help.

Understanding Post-Traumatic Stress Disorder

You feel agitated and keyed up. Were you also exposed to a traumatic event that resulted as follows?

>> At the time, you felt helpless and afraid.

>> Later, you try not to think about it.

>> In spite of your efforts not to think about it, the thoughts and images keep on popping up.

If so, you may have *post-traumatic stress disorder* (PTSD). The treatment of PTSD is probably best done by an experienced professional. Many people with PTSD try to tough it out and live life less fully because of their stubbornness.

Going through Sleepless Nights

Is anxiety keeping you awake? That's quite common. If your sleep doesn't improve after working on your anxiety awhile, be sure to read Chapter 11 about sleep. Too many sleepless nights make it hard to function and more difficult to help yourself in the fight against anxiety. If you sleep poorly night after night and awaken tired, check it out with a professional. You may be experiencing depression along with anxiety. Furthermore, insomnia is a treatable condition by professionals.

Getting High

Sure, a beer or three can seemingly soothe the soul, but excessive drinking or drug abuse is a common problem among those with anxiety disorders. It makes sense; anxious feelings are uncomfortable. What begins as an innocent attempt at feeling better can become another big problem later on. If you find yourself consuming too much alcohol or another drug to calm your feelings, get professional help before the crutch turns into an addiction.

Finding Help

In the days of high-cost healthcare, you may not always have as much freedom to consult any professional you want. However, whether you receive a restricted list of professionals from your insurance company or not, it's still a good idea to check out one or more of the following:

>> Ask the insurance company or the state licensing board for the specific profession or license of the referred professional.

>> Ask your friends if they know of someone whom they had a good experience with.

>> Ask your primary care provider. Family physicians usually have a good idea about excellent referrals for various types of problems.

>> Talk to the professional before making an appointment. Ask about his experience with treating anxiety and what approach he takes. Ask about whether you'll receive a scientifically verified approach for dealing with anxiety.

>> Call the psychology department of your local college or university. Sometimes they have referral lists.

>> Call or use a search engine on the web to find your state psychological, psychiatric, or counseling association. Or, check out national consumer organizations. (See the appendix in the back of this book for more information.)

Resources for You

In this appendix, we provide some books and websites about anxiety for adults and kids as well as some books about racism that embellish our chapter on racism and anxiety. These are only a few of the many excellent resources available to supplement information in this book.

Books about Anxiety

Anxiety & Depression Workbook For Dummies, by Charles Elliott and Laura Smith (Wiley)

The Anxiety and Phobia Workbook, by Edmund Bourne (New Harbinger Publications)

Changing for Good: The Revolutionary Program that Explains the Six Stages of Change and Teaches You How to Free Yourself from Bad Habits, by James Prochaska, John Norcross, and Carlo DiClemente (William Morrow & Co., Inc.)

The Feeling Good Handbook, by David Burns (Plume)

Get Out of Your Mind & Into Your Life: The New Acceptance and Commitment Therapy, by Steven Hayes (New Harbinger Publications)

Mastery of Your Anxiety and Worry: Workbook (Treatments That Work), by Michelle Craske and David Barlow (Oxford University Press, USA)

Mind Over Mood: Change How You Feel by Changing the Way You Think, by Dennis Greenberger and Christine Padesky (The Guilford Press)

The Anxiety & Worry Workbook: The Cognitive Behavioral Solution, by David A. Clark and Aaron T. Beck (The Guilford Press)

The Shyness & Social Anxiety Workbook: Proven, Step-by-Step Techniques for Overcoming Your Fear, by Martin Antony and Richard Swinson (New Harbinger Publications)

The Worry Cure: Seven Steps to Stop Worry from Stopping You, by Robert Leahy (Three Rivers Press)

Books about Racism

Begin Again: James Baldwin's America and Its Urgent Lessons for Our Own, by Eddie S. Glaude Jr. (Crown)

How to Be an Antiracist, by Ibram X. Kendi (One World)

So You Want to Talk About Race, by Ijeoma Oluo (Seal Press)

Stamped from the Beginning: The Definitive History of Racist Ideas in America, by Ibram X. Kendi (Bold Type Books)

Tears We Cannot Stop: A Sermon to White America, by Michael Eric Dyson (St. Martin's Press)

The New Jim Crow: Mass Incarceration in the Age of Colorblindness, by Michelle Alexander (The New Press)

White Fragility: Why It's So Hard for White People to Talk About Racism, by Robin DiAngelo (Beacon Press)

Resources to Help Anxious Children

Cat's Got Your Tongue? A Story for Children Afraid to Speak, by Charles Schaefer (Magination Press)

My Anxious Mind: A Teen's Guide to Managing Anxiety and Panic, by Michael Tompkins and Katherine Martinez (Magination Press)

Outsmarting Worry: An Older Kid's Guide to Managing Anxiety, by Dawn Huebner (Jessica Kingsley Publishers)

The Worry Workbook for Kids: Helping Children to Overcome Anxiety and the Fear of Uncertainty, by Muniya S. Khanna and Deborah Roth Ledley (New Harbinger Publications)

Wemberly Worried, by Kevin Henkes (Harper Collins)

What to Do When You Worry Too Much: A Kid's Guide to Overcoming Anxiety, by Dawn Huebner (Magination Press)

Websites to Discover More about Anxiety

WARNING

Type the word "anxiety" into a search engine, and literally thousands of sites pop up. Be careful. The web is full of unscrupulous sales pitches and misinformation. Be especially cautious about official-sounding organizations that promote materials for sale. Don't be fooled by instant cures for anxiety.

Many web forums host chat rooms for persons with anxiety concerns. Feel free to access them for support.

WARNING

At the same time, realize that you don't know who's sitting on the other end. They may be uneducated about anxiety or, worse, trying to take advantage of a person in distress. Don't believe everything you read.

Here's a list of a variety of legitimate websites that don't sell snake oil:

>> **The American Psychiatric Association** (www.psychiatry.org/patients-families) has information for the public about anxiety and other mental disorders.

>> **The American Psychological Association** (www.apa.org/helpcenter) provides information to the public about treatment and interesting facts about anxiety and other emotional disorders.

>> **The Anxiety and Depression Association of America** (www.adaa.org) lists self-help groups across the United States. They also display a variety of anxiety screening tools for self-assessment. On their site you can find an online newsletter and a message board.

>> **The Association for Behavioral and Cognitive Therapies** (www.abct.org) is a large professional organization that focuses on research-validated treatment approaches for people with emotional disorders. We often refer people to their extensive list of qualified therapists.

>> **The National Alliance on Mental Illness** (www.nami.org) is a wonderful organization that serves as an advocate for people and families affected by mental disorders. Information is available about causes, prevalence, and treatments of disorders for children and adults. This group also offers support groups across the country.

>> **The National Institute of Mental Health** (www.nimh.nih.gov) reports on research about a wide variety of mental health issues. It also has an array of educational materials on anxiety. It provides resources for researchers and practitioners in the field.

Index

A

acceptance. *See also* mindful acceptance
  of anxiety, 313, 317
  of anxiety in loved ones, 279–280
  of discomfort and distress, 141–142
  self-acceptance, 49–51
  of uncertainty and risk
    of danger and trauma, 261–264
    mindful acceptance and, 126–127
    of natural disasters, 233
    during pandemic, 211
acceptance and commitment therapy (ACT), 61
ACE (angiotensin-converting enzyme) inhibitors, 40
action stage of change, 56
active coping, 236–237
addiction to medication, 156, 162, 312
adversity, finding silver lining in, 231–232
agoraphobia
  coaching process for, 276–278
  COVID-19 pandemic and, 153
  in *DSM-5*, 23
  general discussion, 26–27
air pollution, COVID-19 infection and, 229
alcohol, drinking before sleeping, 185
alcohol abuse
  anxiety as risk factor for, 41, 311
  benzodiazepines and, 162
  blocking emotions with, 70
  professional help for, seeking, 322–323
  withdrawal symptoms, 32
allies to people of color, becoming, 251–252
all-or-none words, 95, 96–97, 100
American Psychiatric Association, 327
American Psychological Association, 327
angiotensin-converting enzyme (ACE) inhibitors, 40
antidepressants, 159–161
antihistamines, 40
anxiety

benefits of, 18–20
books about, 325
caused by treating anxiety, 311
costs of, 9–10
famous people who struggled with, 50
rising rates of, 8
roots of, 46–49
Anxiety and Depression Association of America, 327
anxiety disorders
  agoraphobia
    coaching process for, 276–278
    COVID-19 pandemic and, 153
    in *DSM-5*, 23
    general discussion, 26–27
  brain circuits involved in, 34
  in DSM-5, 23
  emotional disorders versus, 30–32
  excessive worry, 20–21
  overview, 17–18
  panic attacks
    description of, 8
    exercise and, 182
    experiencing sensations of, 152–153
    exposure for, 151–153
    general discussion, 24–26
    mistaken for heart attacks, 26
    self-acceptance, 51
  phobias
    avoidance of, 12
    in children, 286–287
    exposure for, 150–151
    general discussion, 27–29
    inoculating children against, 294–295
    school, 283, 285
    types of, 13
  racism-related anxiety versus, 247
  selective mutism, 29
  separation anxiety, 29, 284–286
  social anxiety, 22–24

B

baby steps to change, 54–55

balance sheet, financial, 218–220

balanced assumptions, developing

  for dependency, 120–121

  for need for approval, 118–119

  for need for control, 120

  overview, 116–117

  for perfectionism, 117–118

  for vulnerability, 119

balanced views card, 117

behavior, anxious

  avoidance

    accepting discomfort and distress, 141–142

    breaking cycle of, 140–141

    emotional, 138

    ineffectiveness of, 309

    obvious strategies, 139

    overview, 11–12, 137–138

    subtle strategies, 139–140

  driven by emotions, 68

  overview, 14

behavior therapy (BT), 15, 61

being kind to yourself, 121, 127–128

benzodiazepines, 40, 162–163

beta blockers, 40, 163

biases, cognitive, 209–210

biological roots of anxiety

  anxiety-mimicking drugs, 39–40

  brain connections and neurotransmitters, 33–36

  diet, 41

  fight-or-flight response, 36–37

  freeze response, 37–38

  medical conditions, 42–43

bipolar disorder, 31

black-or-white words, 96–97, 100

Blacks, racism against

  allies, becoming, 251–252

  anxiety caused by, 244, 246–247

  blatant and subtle messages, 240–241

  books about, 326

  colorism, 245

  coping with, 244, 248–251

  covert, 243–245

  educating children about, 253

  emotions, expressing, 250

  empowerment, finding, 249

  exposure to minorities, increasing, 253

  fighting, 251–253

  internalized, 245

  interpersonal, 243–245

  overt, 243

  overview, 239–240

  public racism examples, 246–247

  self-care, 250

  self-education, 252

  speaking up against, 252–253

  staying connected, 249–250

  structural, 241–243

  teen drivers, parental anxiety for, 19

  Windrush scandal, 242

blame, avoiding, 271

body scan meditation, 193–194

books, recommended, 325–326

booster sessions, 316

Boston Molasses Tragedy, 263

brain

  circuit connections, 34

  fight-or-flight response, 36–37

  freeze response, 37–38

  neurotransmitters, 34, 35–36, 293

  overview, 33–34

brain stimulation techniques, 170–171

breathing meditation, 192–193

British Medical Journal, 35

bronchodilators, 40

BT (behavior therapy), 15, 61

budgeting, 219–220

Buspar (buspirone), 163

C

caffeine, 40, 41, 185

calm thinking, cultivating, 91–94

calm view of anxiety, taking, 124–126

calming anxious children, 294

cancer, fear of, 88–90

cannabidiol (CBD), 168

carbon footprint, reducing, 237

cardiovascular disease, 9
career-related anxiety
  careers with stability, considering, 216–217
  flexibility, importance of, 215–216
  keeping focused, 217–218
  overview, 214
  resumes, writing, 214–215
  retirement planning, 223
  searching for jobs, 221–222
CBD (cannabidiol), 168
CBT (cognitive behavior therapy), 61
change process
  excuses for not changing, 51–53
  goals in, working towards, 54–55
  ineffective approaches, 309–312
  origins of anxiety, 46–49
  positive psychology, importance of, 58
  relapses, dealing with, 313–317
  self-acceptance, 49–51
  stages in, 56
  staying motivated, 53–56
  tracking anxiety levels, 57–60
children
  assumptions, acquisition of, 109
  Black teen drivers, anxiety about, 19
  comforting reassurance, resisting desire to give, 295–296
  early mastery experiences, 292
  educating about racism, 253
  emotional management, 293–294
  excessive worry about, exposure process for, 148–150
  exercise for anxiety, 301–302
  exposure strategies for, 300–301
  generalized anxiety in, 286
  helping anxious, 298–302, 326
  modeling mellow for, 299
  normal versus abnormal anxiety in, 282–284
  OCD in, 287
  parenting styles, role in anxiety, 46, 47–48, 296–298
  parent's anxiety, effect on, 10
  phobias of, 286–287, 294–295
  PTSD in, 288
  school phobia in, 283, 285–286
  selective mutism in, 29
  separation anxiety in, 29, 284–286
  silent anxiety in, 289

  sleep disorders in, 283
  social fears in, 288
  therapy for, 303–305
Chinese handcuffs, 124
cholinergic system, 35
chronic anxiety, impact on health, 9, 37, 38
chronic lung conditions, 43
church membership, 250
circuits, brain, 34
climate change, assessing risks from, 229
coaching process, 274–278
cognitive behavior therapy (CBT), 61
cognitive biases, 209–210
cognitive dissonance, 210
cognitive therapy (CT), 14–15, 60–61
collaborating with loved ones to reduce stress, 278–279
colorism, 245
comforting reassurance, 295–296, 310
commandments
  identifying, 95, 97–98
  replacing, 100–101
communication
  coaching process, 274–278
  silent anxiety in children, 289
  support groups, 315–316
  talking with loved ones about anxiety, 269–273
community
  staying connected to, 176–178, 208
  support for coping with racism, 249–250
  volunteering, 236, 237, 278
complaining, 310
compulsions, 287, 321–322
concentration problems, 11
concern, expressing, 271
Confederate flag, 243
confidence killers, 49
confirmation bias, 209
connecting with others
  coping with racism, 249–250
  importance of, 176–178
  during pandemic, 208
  support groups, 315–316
contemplation stage of change, 56
control assumption
  assessing, 106–108
  balancing, 120

EPS (extrapyramidal side effects), 164
evidence for anxious thoughts, searching for, 80, 81–83
evidence-based treatment, 259
evidence-gathering questions, 81–83
excessive worry
  exposure for, 148–150
  general discussion, 20–21
excuses for not seeking help, 51–53
exercise
  anxiety reduced with, 178–179
  as daily goal during pandemic, 207
  encouraging in children, 301–302
  gym memberships, saving money on, 220
  with loved ones suffering anxiety, 278
  motivation for, 180–181
  panic attacks and, 182
  scheduling, 181–182
expenses, cutting, 218, 219–220
exposure
  for children, 300–301
  coaching process, 274–278
  for excessive worry, 148–150
  for fear of natural disasters, 235–236
  list of goals, constructing, 145–146
  overcoming anxiety, 153–154
  overview, 15, 142–143
  for panic attacks, 151–153
  for phobias, 150–151
  procedures, 146–148
  relapse, dealing with, 316
  tips for, 147
  understanding fears, 143–145
exposure to minorities, increasing, 253
extrapyramidal side effects (EPS), 164
extremist words, 95–96, 99

F

fake news, identifying, 209–210
family. See also children; parents
  accepting anxiety in members of, 279–280
  coaching process, 274–278
  coping with racism, support from, 249–250
  discerning anxiety in, 268–270
  reassurance requests, responding to, 271–273

relationship counseling, 270
spending time with, 176–178
staying connected during pandemic, 208
stress, collaborating to reduce, 278–279
talking together about anxiety, 269–273
famous people who struggled with anxiety, 50
fat, effect of anxiety on, 10
fears. See also specific types
  avoidance, 137–140
  common, 30
  coping questions, 87, 88–89
  exposure procedures, 153–154
  phobias
    avoidance, 12, 137–140
    in children, 286–287
    exposure for, 150–151
    general discussion, 27–29
    inoculating children against, 294–295
    school, 283, 285
    types of, 13
  risk, calculating odds of, 83–85
  ultimate coping questions, 90–91
  understanding, 143–145
Feeling Cycle Chart, 76–77
feeling symptoms, 14
feelings
  behavior driven by, 68
  blocking, 69–70
  caused by racism, expressing, 250
  control of, teaching to children, 293–294
  defining, 66
  "don't feel" messages, 70
  Feeling Cycle Chart, 76–77
  hiding, reasons behind, 268
  hopelessness, 320
  identifying, 70–72
  list of anxious, 72
  overview, 65–66
  physical sensations from, 67–68
  primary six, 66
  role of, 67
  suppressing, 250
  thoughts, influence on, 68–69
  triggers, understanding, 73–74
  trouble identifying, 69–70

household chores (during pandemic), 208

hurricanes, 227, 229, 288

hyperthyroidism, 43

hypoglycemia, 43

I

IBS (irritable bowel syndrome), 42

icons, used in book, 2–3

imaginal exposure, 235–236. *See also* exposure

imperfections, appreciating, 128–130

inconsistent responders, 48

indigenous people, racism against, 248

infection, vulnerability to, 35

insomnia, 186–187, 191, 322

instant gratification, 310

internalized racism, 245

interpersonal racism, 243–245

irritable bowel syndrome (IBS), 42

J

job worries

careers with stability, considering, 216–217

flexibility, importance of, 215–216

keeping focused, 217–218

overview, 214

resumes, writing, 214–215

retirement planning, 223

searching for jobs, 221–222

journaling

Appreciating Flawed Friends exercise, 129–130

arguments against excuses for staying stuck, 53–54

benefits of, 59

Feeling Cycle Chart, 76–77

positive emotions, 58, 59–60

positive psychology, importance of, 58

reasonable perspective, developing calm thoughts with, 92–94

tracking anxiety levels, 57–58

what to include, 59

judging words

identifying, 95, 97–98

replacing, 100–101

K

kava kava, 167

L

labels

identifying, 95, 97–98

replacing, 100–101

law enforcement careers, 217

liabilities, personal, 218–221

lifestyle. *See also* meditation

daily goals during pandemic, 207–208

diet

emotional eating, 187

healthy eating during pandemic, 208

nutrition, 188

portion sizes, 188

tasting meditation, 194–195

unhealthy foods and substances, 41

exercise

anxiety reduced with, 178–179

as daily goal during pandemic, 207

encouraging in children, 301–302

gym memberships, saving money on, 220

with loved ones suffering anxiety, 278

motivation for, 180–181

panic attacks and, 182

friends and family, spending time with, 176–178

overview, 15, 175

sleep

childhood disorders, 283

insomnia, 186–187, 191, 322

medications, impact on, 186

overview, 182–183

physical environment, preparing for, 183–184

problems with, 186–187

relaxing routines for, 184–186

limbic system, 34

living in future and predicting the worst, 11

London Beer Flood of 1814, 263

losing job, fear of. *See* job worries

N

naps, 187
narrative bias, 210
National Alliance on Mental Illness, 327
National Institute of Mental Health, 327
natural disasters
    active coping, 236–237
    adversity, finding silver lining in, 231–232
    anxiety due to, 49
    climate change, assessing risks from, 229
    coping ability, evaluating, 233–235
    exposure strategy, 235–236
    helping with environment, 237
    impact on children, 288
    likelihood of dying from, 226–228
    overview, 225–226
    personal risks, calculating, 228–229
    preparing plan for, 230–231
    risk, assessing, 226–229
    risk of death, evaluating, 255–256
    uncertainty and risk, accepting, 233
    volunteering after disasters, 237
neurons, 34
neurotransmitters, 34, 35–36, 293
news
    anxiety due to, 8, 208
    fake news, identifying, 209–210
nicotine, 185
Niebuhr, Reinhold, 135
"no", learning to say, 177–178
noradrenergic system, 35
normal versus abnormal anxiety in children, 282–284
notebooks, writing in. *See* journaling
novocaine, 40
nutrition, 188. *See also* diet

O

objectively observing anxiety, 124–126
obsessions, 287, 321–322
obsessive-compulsive disorder (OCD)
    in children, 287
    in *DSM-5*, 23
    general discussion, 30–31
    seeking help for, 321–322

Occupational Outlook Handbook, 217
odds of unwanted events, recalculating, 83–85
Omega-3 fatty acids, 169
online courses, 216
origins of anxiety, 46–49
over-controllers, 48
overestimating odds, 83–85
overprotecting children, 47–48, 294
overt racism, 243

P

pandemic-related anxiety
    accepting emotions, 203–204
    air pollution, COVID-19 infection and, 229
    daily goals, setting, 207–208
    denying risks of pandemic, 203
    emergency supplies, gathering, 206–207
    fake news, identifying, 209–210
    hoarding of toilet paper, 205
    job worries, 214–218
    overview, 49, 201–202
    personal safety decisions, 211–212
    staying connected, 208
    uncertainty of future, dealing with, 211
    useful versus useless, 204–206
    wallowing response, 203–204
panic attacks
    description of, 8
    exercise and, 182
    experiencing sensations of, 152–153
    exposure for, 151–153
    general discussion, 24–26
    mistaken for heart attacks, 26
    self-acceptance, 51
panic disorder, 24–26
parenting styles
    authoritarian, 296–297
    authoritative, 297
    helicopter parenting, 298
    overview, 296
    permissive, 296–297
    role in anxiety, 46, 47–48

for racism-related anxiety, 247
relapse, dealing with, 314, 316
seeking right therapies, 60–61
seeking right therapists, 61–62
staying motivated to change, 53–56
protests, participating in, 249, 250
psychoanalysis, 312
psychosis, 31–32
PTSD (post-traumatic stress disorder)
in children, 288
in *DSM-5*, 23
general discussion, 31, 158
seeking help for, 260, 322

Q

questions
coping
for cancer anxiety, 88–89
for fear of earthquakes, 234–235
for fear of flying, 90–91
for job loss anxiety, 87–88
evidence-gathering, 81–83
minding-your-mind, 75–76
reassessment of risk, 83–85
talking with loved ones about anxiety, 269–270
quick fixes for emotional upsets, 310

R

racing thoughts, 11
racism
allies, becoming, 251–252
anxiety caused by, 246–247
Black teen drivers, anxiety about, 19
blatant and subtle messages, 240–241
books about, 326
colorism, 245
coping with, 244, 248–251
covert, 243–245
educating children about, 253
emotions, expressing, 250
empowerment, finding, 249
exposure to minorities, increasing, 253
family physician's perspective on, 244

fighting, 251–253
against First peoples, 248
internalized, 245
interpersonal, 243–245
overt, 243
overview, 239–240
self-care, 250
self-education, 252
speaking up against, 252–253
staying connected, 249–250
structural, 241–243
Windrush scandal, 242
rare anxiety disorders, 29
reasonable perspective, developing calm thoughts with, 92–94
reassessment of risk questions, 83–85
reassurance requests, responding to, 271–273, 295–296
Red Cross, 237
relapses, dealing with, 313–317
relationships. *See* family; friends; partners with anxiety
relaxing routines for sleep, 184–186
religion, 250
Remember icon, 2
repetition bias, 209
repression of emotions, 70
resilience, 46, 251
resources
books, 325–326
meditation, 197
websites, 327
resources, personal, 218–221
resumes, writing, 214–215
retirement planning, 223
reward system for exercising, 180–181
risks
of anxious thoughts coming true, recalculating, 80, 83–85
avoiding unnecessary, 257–259
danger, accepting, 261–264
of death, 255–256
high-risk jobs, 261–262
of natural disasters, 226–229, 233
personal, evaluating, 255–256
Roosevelt, Eleanor, 50
roots of anxiety, 46–49

Notes

Notes

About the Authors

Drs. Smith and Elliott are clinical psychologists who have worked on numerous publications together. They are coauthors of *Quitting Smoking & Vaping For Dummies* (Wiley); *Anger Management For Dummies* (Wiley); *Borderline Personality Disorder For Dummies* (Wiley); *Child Psychology & Development For Dummies* (Wiley); *Obsessive Compulsive Disorder For Dummies* (Wiley); *Seasonal Affective Disorder For Dummies* (Wiley); *Anxiety & Depression Workbook For Dummies* (Wiley); *Depression For Dummies* (Wiley); *Hollow Kids: Recapturing the Soul of a Generation Lost to the Self-Esteem Myth* (Prima Lifestyles); and *Why Can't I Be the Parent I Want to Be?* (New Harbinger). They have committed their professional lives to making the science of psychology relevant and accessible to the public.

Authors' Acknowledgments

We want to thank our outstanding team at Wiley. As usual, their expertise, support, and guidance was of immeasurable help. From the beginning, our acquisition editor, Kelsey Baird, helped us formulate and execute a plan for developing *Anxiety For Dummies*. Tim Gallan, masterful project editor, ensured that our text stayed coherent and on point. We also thank Joseph Bush, our technical editor, for his contributions.

Special thanks to Latasha Seliby Perkins, MD, member of the board of American Academy of Family Physicians, for her astute insight and advice for the chapter on anxiety and racism.

Publisher's Acknowledgments

Acquisitions Editor: Kelsey Baird

Project Editor: Tim Gallan

Copy Editor: Christine Pingleton

Technical Reviewer: Joseph P. Bush, PhD

Production Editor: Mohammed Zafar Ali

Cover Image: © Peter Cade/Getty Images

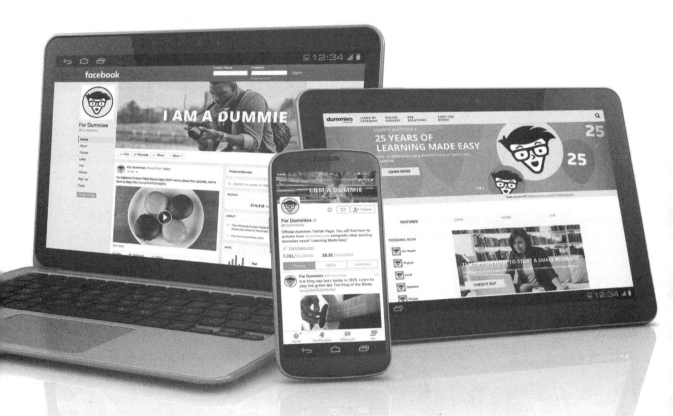
  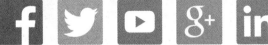
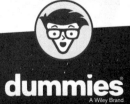

Leverage the power

Dummies is the global leader in the reference category and one of the most trusted and highly regarded brands in the world. No longer just focused on books, customers now have access to the dummies content they need in the format they want. Together we'll craft a solution that engages your customers, stands out from the competition, and helps you meet your goals.

Advertising & Sponsorships

Connect with an engaged audience on a powerful multimedia site, and position your message alongside expert how-to content. Dummies.com is a one-stop shop for free, online information and know-how curated by a team of experts.

- Targeted ads
- Video
- Email Marketing
- Microsites
- Sweepstakes sponsorship

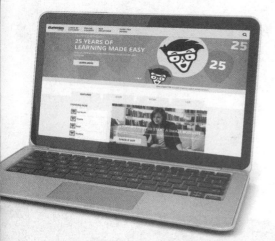

20 MILLION PAGE VIEWS **EVERY SINGLE MONTH**

15 MILLION UNIQUE VISITORS PER MONTH

43% OF ALL VISITORS ACCESS THE SITE **VIA THEIR MOBILE DEVICES**

700,000 NEWSLETTER SUBSCRIPTIONS **TO THE INBOXES OF** *300,000* UNIQUE INDIVIDUALS EVERY WEEK

# of dummies

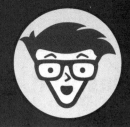

Custom Publishing

Reach a global audience in any language by creating a solution that will differentiate you from competitors, amplify your message, and encourage customers to make a buying decision.

- Apps
- Books
- eBooks
- Video
- Audio
- Webinars

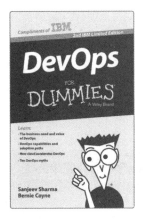

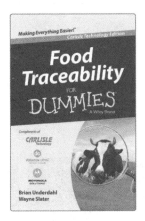

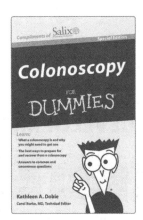

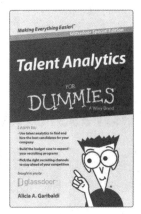

Brand Licensing & Content

Leverage the strength of the world's most popular reference brand to reach new audiences and channels of distribution.

For more information, visit dummies.com/biz

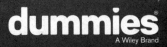

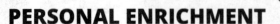

PERSONAL ENRICHMENT

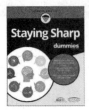
Staying Sharp
9781119187790
USA $26.00
CAN $31.99
UK £19.99

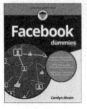
Facebook
9781119179030
USA $21.99
CAN $25.99
UK £16.99

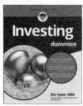
Guitar
9781119293354
USA $24.99
CAN $29.99
UK £17.99

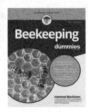
Investing
9781119293347
USA $22.99
CAN $27.99
UK £16.99

Beekeeping
9781119310068
USA $22.99
CAN $27.99
UK £16.99

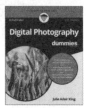
Digital Photography
9781119235606
USA $24.99
CAN $29.99
UK £17.99

Meditation
9781119251163
USA $24.99
CAN $29.99
UK £17.99

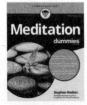
Pregnancy All-in-One
9781119235491
USA $26.99
CAN $31.99
UK £19.99

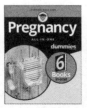
Samsung Galaxy S7
9781119279952
USA $24.99
CAN $29.99
UK £17.99

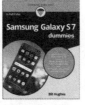
iPhone
9781119283133
USA $24.99
CAN $29.99
UK £17.99

Crocheting
9781119287117
USA $24.99
CAN $29.99
UK £16.99

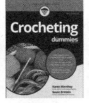
Nutrition
9781119130246
USA $22.99
CAN $27.99
UK £16.99

PROFESSIONAL DEVELOPMENT

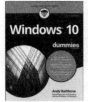
Windows 10
9781119311041
USA $24.99
CAN $29.99
UK £17.99

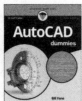
AutoCAD
9781119255796
USA $39.99
CAN $47.99
UK £27.99

Excel 2016
9781119293439
USA $26.99
CAN $31.99
UK £19.99

QuickBooks 2017
9781119281467
USA $26.99
CAN $31.99
UK £19.99

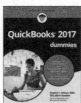
macOS Sierra
9781119280651
USA $29.99
CAN $35.99
UK £21.99

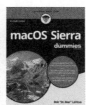
LinkedIn
9781119251132
USA $24.99
CAN $29.99
UK £17.99

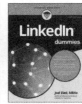
Windows 10 All-in-One
9781119310563
USA $34.00
CAN $41.99
UK £24.99

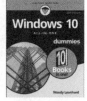
SharePoint 2016
9781119181705
USA $29.99
CAN $35.99
UK £21.99

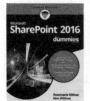
Fundamental Analysis
9781119263593
USA $26.99
CAN $31.99
UK £19.99

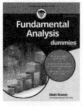
Networking
9781119257769
USA $29.99
CAN $35.99
UK £21.99

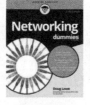
Office 2016
9781119293477
USA $26.99
CAN $31.99
UK £19.99

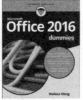
Office 365
9781119265313
USA $24.99
CAN $29.99
UK £17.99

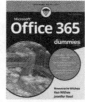
Salesforce.com
9781119239314
USA $29.99
CAN $35.99
UK £21.99

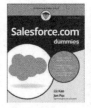
Coding
9781119293323
USA $29.99
CAN $35.99
UK £21.99

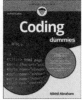

dummies.com

dummies
A Wiley Brand

Learning Made Easy

ACADEMIC

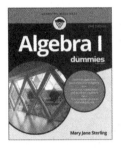

9781119293576
USA $19.99
CAN $23.99
UK £15.99

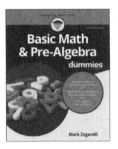

9781119293637
USA $19.99
CAN $23.99
UK £15.99

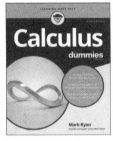

9781119293491
USA $19.99
CAN $23.99
UK £15.99

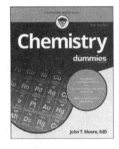

9781119293460
USA $19.99
CAN $23.99
UK £15.99

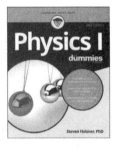

9781119293590
USA $19.99
CAN $23.99
UK £15.99

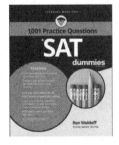

9781119215844
USA $26.99
CAN $31.99
UK £19.99

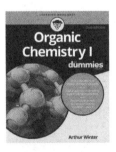

9781119293378
USA $22.99
CAN $27.99
UK £16.99

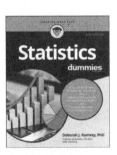

9781119293521
USA $19.99
CAN $23.99
UK £15.99

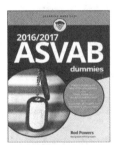

9781119239178
USA $18.99
CAN $22.99
UK £14.99

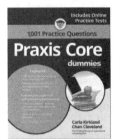

9781119263883
USA $26.99
CAN $31.99
UK £19.99

Available Everywhere Books Are Sold

dummies.com

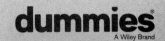

Small books for big imaginations

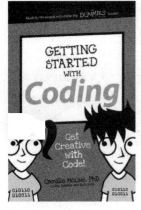

GETTING STARTED WITH **Coding**

Get Creative with Code!

Camille McCue, PhD

9781119177173
USA $9.99
CAN $9.99
UK £8.99

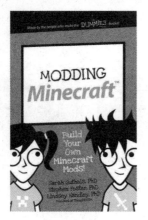

MODDING **Minecraft**™

Build Your Own Minecraft Mods!

Sarah Guthals, PhD
Stephen Foster, PhD
Lindsey Handley, PhD

9781119177272
USA $9.99
CAN $9.99
UK £8.99

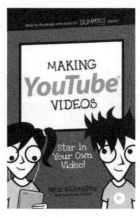

MAKING **YouTube** VIDEOS

Star in Your Own Video!

Nick Willoughby

9781119177241
USA $9.99
CAN $9.99
UK £8.99

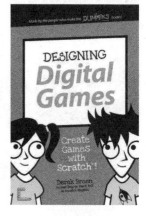

DESIGNING **Digital Games**

Create Games with Scratch™!

Derek Breen

9781119177210
USA $9.99
CAN $9.99
UK £8.99

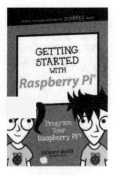

GETTING STARTED WITH **Raspberry Pi**®

Program Your Raspberry Pi!

Richard Wentk

9781119262657
USA $9.99
CAN $9.99
UK £6.99

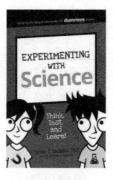

EXPERIMENTING WITH **Science**

Think, Test, and Learn!

9781119291336
USA $9.99
CAN $9.99
UK £6.99

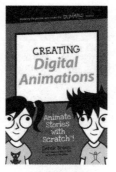

CREATING **Digital Animations**

Animate Stories with Scratch™!

Derek Breen

9781119233527
USA $9.99
CAN $9.99
UK £6.99

GETTING STARTED WITH **Engineering**

Think Like an Engineer!

Camille McCue, PhD

9781119291220
USA $9.99
CAN $9.99
UK £6.99

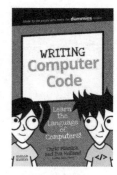

WRITING **Computer Code**

Learn the Language of Computers!

Chris Minnick
and Eva Holland

9781119177302
USA $9.99
CAN $9.99
UK £8.99

Unleash Their Creativity

dummies.com

dummies®
A Wiley Brand